Spot a Liar

A Practical Guide to Speed Read People

(How to Learn the Parts of the Brain That Are Important to the Lie)

Darnell Benjamin

Published By **John Kembrey**

Darnell Benjamin

Spot a Liar: A Practical Guide to Speed Read People (How to Learn the Parts of the Brain That Are Important to the Lie)

ISBN   978-1-7774403-6-7

No part of this guidebook shall be reproduced in any form without permission in writing from the publisher except in the case of brief quotations embodied in critical articles or reviews.

Legal & Disclaimer

Table Of Contents

Chapter 1: How To Appear Strong

Dominant Body Language

A common form of non-verbal communication could be confused by forceful non-verbal messages. The active hips make the elbows expand and makes people's bodies seem larger and in addition, when a person is standing upright, with their midsection extended and their jaw pointing upwards. The height is also important because it allows individuals a choice when there is the possibility of ambush. A different indicator of strength could be intrusion in the domain of an individual who can have a superior one. in this way be standing with their feet firm and firmly positioned with hips. Rulers do not have to follow the lead of their principles. They set their own standards. Your ability to make decisions in the way you want to go may lead you to break norms of social behavior. If you possess something other people wish you had, this creates the impression of status. It suggests that when you own something that other people consider to be superior or a high level of support, there are people who try to show the item, such as the Rolex timepiece, a display of wealth, or even employing workers. If you own these types of objects, when used in non-verbal communicating, it's an expression of strength in the event that you show your pictures. Another common practice is attacking another's space through excessively close proximity to the person and generally slapping their privacy. Other actions include placing your feet over the other person's side table, occupying seats with a different individual or a significant over-accommodation with their partner. The person who is the most popular will begin with higher standing positions in which they will be noticed by others. In the event that the table's rectangular they'll sit towards the top or take a seat in the corner.

The group will also remain within the crowd and be able to stand back from others (however they won't be afraid to the possibility of a strike). They'll also stroll through the middle of a path or walkway and hope that other people will get out of their way. The arrangements for moving on start at a distance, and they proceed without making any movements in order for others to make.

The majority of people will want at ways to limit time more. When they are in discussions in which they are able to be more vocal and block other participants time to discuss such as by interfering or announcing their departure early. A different strategy is to hurry or talking quickly while making sure to check the time and then asking others to remain brief. In the absence of discussion it is possible that they are not available when you need however, you can ask your immediate attention. Signs of superiority are found when you say 'I'm important', and also "you're not important". Then, a person who is overwhelmed may be unable to see or hear the other person conversing or deflecting their surroundings. They might scold the weak one, and even when they can be heard. They might examine their nails or generally show no focus on the other person. A general trim can also indicate lack of appreciation. The act of pressing the button demonstrates judgement.

A lot of strength could be seen through the eyes by a variety of expressions, from scowls at each other and lips that are pressed inwards to growls and jeers (some times time concealed as grins). Eyes can be used to focus and keep the gaze for an extended period of time. You may also squint while keeping the other person from seeing the area you're looking at. It is also possible to look around and the other party is able to say that they don't even have anything worthy of looking at'. A squinty eye indicates suspicion, perhaps even aversion. People who confront each other may look tired and smug or have diverse interpretations, which denigrate each other. Heads do nothing at all. One of the most effective tricks is to keep the head in a fixed position. People tend to move their heads while they speak and interact with other people. The way we look at the behavior of people around us. The extraordinary layout and a calm in the face and head indicate comfort and peace. Most people smile a lot, and are not necessarily resigned people. Handshakes are best done using the palm downwards, usually on one side. Another popular handshake is for a pounding on the opponent.

Handing someone else's longer than normal shows that you're in the control.

Unblinking, delaying eye contact can be interpreted as exaggerating handshakes and demonstrates that 'I'm adept, I'm able to defy the laws.' A majority of people however be anticipating eye contact to say that "you're beneath me, and I'm not even required to look at your face.' One who speaks most often is the one who controls the conversation either through a lengthy discussion or addressing the questions. In the event that other people display an unspoken communication, you are presented with many options.

The most straightforward response is not to give in and that is something they're likely to would like to do. Maintain a friendly appearance and ignore their subtle signs.

Another option is to fight strength by the dominant position, such as:

You can out-gaze them (a way to gaze at the slats of their noses, not the eyes).

You can touch them before they get close to you, or as they come in contact with you.

If they make a strong handshake, grab their wrist and walk towards the other side.

If they interrupt your conversation speed up, speak with more ferocity and say, "Let me get to the end and then let me finish!'

Another option is to mention the entertainment. Find out the reason they're engaging in non-verbal communications.

Aggressive Body Language

Body language that is aggressive is a sign of an inclination to a physical threat, or threats verbally. Being aware of and recognizing signals could lead to either you reverting back to your body language in a hostile manner and that's not an ideal thing, and nothing benefit is gained and you could reduce the aggressive behavior before any other thing happens. There are a variety of methods to detect threatening body language, which is caused by attacks, exposure, and face-related aspects.

Let's first discuss the facial features. Take note of the attacker's face, and be conscious of any face signals that could indicate the possibility of a danger. Be aware of frowns, tight pursed lips, a redness on the face, a clenched jaw and squinting eyes, shaking of the head, a snooping of the space, and a smile. No matter what you do, don't give with the same rage towards the person who is at fault because it could be a dangerous concept. One of the best things you could accomplish in this case is take a step back and put some distance from the aggressor.

The stance of attack is well-known by the attacker who positions their feet so that they can remain stable while maintaining their fists tightly clenched. One can determine if someone is in an attack mode simply by looking at their muscles. The attack stance will determine how the opponent is revving up or is ready to combat.

A few clues given could indicate whether someone is dangerous for you. There are times when you will not be able to discern how someone is feeling by the look their expression. It is possible to refer to it as having the poker face. The term refers to the time when someone retains a neutral facial appearance and it is difficult to tell what they're thinking or the way they are feeling. It is possible to find individuals who can be read as if you were reading an open-book. For those who cannot understand, it could be difficult to identify the body language they use. For these types of people, might require you to look for signals in their speech as well as to provide you with any kind of indication that they are not happy with something.

Did you realize that fake friendships can be part of aggressive body language? The fake friendships are only more aggressive when the person who is causing them is attempting to hurt the person. That being said make sure you look out for everything fake, including false smiles, harmful suggestions and anything else that has anything to do with having an effect similar to a chameleon. It is possible that at first, you won't recognize the falsehood, but if you pay attention to indications, the problem will be apparent as it is. A different effect of abusive body language is that it can be seen as invading personal boundaries like physical, mental or emotional limits.

In the event that an aggressor is close to the victim and may cause them to touch the person without consent this is an opportunity to gain influence and control over someone else simply through making them uneasy. If that occurs, the first attack could be made by the attacker and you could become an innocent victim.

Chapter 2: How To Appear Weak

Defensive Body Language

The body language used is utilized for those who are afraid for the purpose of defending their self-defense, whether physical or emotional. Body language that is defensive comes into play when you've experienced school when there was a tornado warning or an alert for hurricanes and the students in the entire class practiced what they should respond to an alert for a tornado. Students take a space with no windows or perhaps some space on the hall and put their heads on the floor. They then cover their head and then crouch in a posture in order to shield vital organs.

In the event that people feel they're about to be threatened or attacked, they are likely to defend their bodies by curling up into a ball and covering their head. They could try looking around the space in search of some escape route could be used because they are afraid at the highest degree.

The barriers are created between an uneasy person and those who pose an obnoxious threat based of defensive body language. In the event that a person feels uncomfortable, they may be unable to communicate with an object, any item they discover, or perhaps someone else.

One of the best ways to determine whether someone is using this kind expression of their body is to to look at their hands. Grips are a crucial way to identify this kind of body expression. In a stressful or difficult situation, gripping is more of a defense mechanism. For women to determine if they have this type of body language it is possible to see them gripping their purse, bag, or bag, and then hold the bag closer to their body. If males exhibit this behavior, they grasp whatever's within their hands, such as keys or even a wallet.

There are some who do not show the signs of defensive body language in the face of threats, therefore they might display more submissive or aggressive body expressions.

Submissive Body Language

Non-verbal communication that is able to be accommodated displays of defeat and is also used to signal fear, which is not to be confused with uninvolved non-verbal communication. Consider a lion who is an lioness. From beginning to end, the lioness is going to fight the beasts to suppress her, and eventually the lion surrenders. She bows in his rage and lets the lion be taken. This is non-verbal docile communication that is prevalent. If there is a signal of anxiety, a person could be pushed in a fetal position, or shut off non-verbal communication until the danger has been eliminated.

One of the most resigned non-verbal signs to look out for are holding the head downwards, not making eyes with people outside or a widening of eyes that appear more blameless as the wide eyes of the eyes of a baby as well as the conscious examination of the eyes of a person who has been speaking to them. This is the primary focus of their attention.

Someone who is friendly will participate with someone who has who has more influence than them but for the greater portion, they'll always agree with their fellows. They'll reach an overwhelming smile, and whatever that their smile will eventually be dispersed. Females tend to be more submissive in verbal communication than males. The males, however, seem to have lost their train of thinking when they conclude that certain females in societies feel resigned by their own nature, such as, Asian ladies.

Asian women aren't much more relaxed than any other women. The culture they live in is unique and they value their families and consider themselves to be an amazing mom and wife. In no way, form or manner will make her hospitable.

Take to the Shadows and Be Hidden

Deceptive Body Language

The deceitful body language can be attributed to be used by those hiding something. What they're hiding could be different from a deceitful lie to an idea, or could be attempting to deceive the victim in some manner either in form or shape. You can tell that someone is trying make fun of you. However, there are those on the planet who have mastered the art of keeping an open poker face while concealing the most outrageous deceit.

They have their entire script in order and are skilled actors. The most effective people with the ability to read deceitful body language include entrepreneurs (who are also known to be extremely clever salespeople) as well as criminals and perhaps even magicians. For those who work in the field of law enforcement are educated to detect deceitful body language in detail, you could be a skilled reader.

First thing to be aware of about deceitful body communication is that it's widely known that when someone intends to appear deceitful, they might look off towards the left. Although this may be the case in certain situations however, it's never correct and shouldn't be relied upon as proof. In some instances, a deceiving person might look at the right side when responding to the question, or even making up an untruth. Looking to the right is a sign of the use of the left part of the brain that used for reasoning and analysis while the right side is utilized to create emotion and imagination. Many scholars believe the left portion of a brain may be utilized to fabricate a falsehood and thus results in eye-gazing towards the right. One reason it's not recommended to utilize eye-gaze analogies to determine deceitful body language is due to the fact that when you are paying attention to anyone when they're in conversation, and you notice that they're trying to recall a particular aspect, they will also exhibit the tendency of looking towards their left to show that they are trying to remember something, so avoid being misled(no pun intended).

Another method to identify fraudulent behaviors is to pay close at the subtle signals such as touching the back of the neck, sweating, intense and body twitches.

Also, you can observe hands in pockets, unexpected movements, sudden changes in the voice and the speed at which speech is spoken. It is possible to observe someone chewing in their mouth, or the most well-known, fidgeting.

A person who willfully deceives might even attempt to maintain in control the way they look and act, changing the way they speak to ensure that it doesn't look suspicious. Some may try to force smiles or hand gestures. One thing you should look out for is the avoidance of eye contact, speaking when not looking at the screen, or even a lack of concentration regardless of whether they are trying to decide what they should say next, or when trying to slow down their speaking speed.

Closed Body Language

The body language of the closed is often displayed by someone who claims that they're listening to you, when actually they're bored of the conversations. They'll allow you to speak and may pretend that they are paying attention, but their body language tells everything. If you asked the person the opportunity to take a quiz right after the discussion, they will be unable to answer and will give the same answer as the following "Well there was something you mentioned regarding ...."

In analyzing this kind of body language, pay close your attention to the eyes of the person. As mentioned in the preceding section Eye contact is crucial. A person who is listening could be a bit distracted, but there are additional signs which you need to be alert for. For instance, distractions are a prime example. When someone gets frequently distracted, despite the fact that they declare that they're listening, the most likely they're not. Only exceptions are when the listener is an excellent multitasker.

The most obvious sign is that you are slouching. If any instructors are who are reading this, the best method to determine closed body language is looking at the signs of the slouching. If someone falls in a state of sleep or begins to drift off while listening to you or conversing with you, the there is a good chance that you need to refresh your present abilities. Another thing to look out for include fidgeting hands eyes, eye-twitching and occasionally eye tearing. If it happens to someone you're communicating with, try not to interpret it as to be personal. The most common reason why a person displays the body is due to what you talk about with them might not seem to necessarily be important, it could be dull or you've had the same conversation time and time. Another reason could be that people get bored easily. Certain people tend to be like this.

In a conversation, it is important to learn how to utilize body language to help get your message through. The use of hand and facial gestures can assist in triggering both audio and visual perceptions in the audience. If hand gestures and facial expressions do not suffice to keep an audience entertained, it's crucial to employ the triple S strategy that is short, sweet and straightforward in addition to quick, sweet and direct. One way to show the audience's interest is to inquire. By asking questions, you can determine the amount of curiosity.

If you have ever spoken to anyone who displays the same body language over and over again, it could be necessary to change the way you talk about a subject. A way of indicating the body is closed if you observe the person is speaking to roll in their heels, then wrap their arms around them, and curled up into the shape of a ball (which is called self-preservation and refers to aggressive behavior due to protecting organs of importance in the event the event of an attachment) however, it is often used to soothe the person) or crossed legs.

The use of closed body language may be used in conjunction with an aggressive tone of voice. For avoiding closed body language, don't assume it's all about your personal style and what you are able to communicate. Also, as the previous point, don't consider it a personal attack. This may not be your presentation abilities. There could be a reason that the person is over the top or had a rough day or feels intimidated (which can be a sign of the defensive or aggressive mode) Or, they might perhaps be hiding some thing. The person may be trying to cover up their emotions such as tears or facial expressions.

The easiest way to help someone from a closed body language and into a more open and accepting body language by giving someone something to hold onto such as something they can place in their hands, for instance a beverage, remote or toy or whatever other than that. If none of that works, it is possible to imitate their body language, but make sure to not use it in a offensive or negative way. It should be gradual. Begin by moving towards the individual, but at a distance that isn't too close. attempt to copy their body expression. This will aid the person in creating a bond that is non-verbal.

Exude Power

Chapter 3: Power Body Language

Force non-verbal communications is an example of a predominant form of non-verbal communications that also includes a heroic or rescue perspective it too. The people who use force non-verbal communication on an overall basis are those who hold a position of authority or prefer to behave as if they believe that they are. There could be a partner or a co-worker who tries to keep the focus on them in the event that someone else uses force communications. If someone appears to be in control of the flow of time as well as space they are more likely to display significant amounts of strategy control of non-verbal communications, and can be confined by that control over your life.

In the world of business, the political influence of the country is exhibited and acknowledged by its representatives, starting at the garage for organizations. People in the positions of power are always in the top stopping places. It is the beginning of controlling space and showing one's position over another. The display shows their location and state from their vehicle as that they travel in to the area of the work area they're within, and an entrance which they are able to close, giving their employees to decide which time to supervise their assistance. They can eat more savoury food items, yet they've got been able to complete the bail punch in order to make sure that they do not exceed the time set by the company.

Handshakes with power are not allowed. person will show their dominance over a different. When they are greeted by someone who whom they think is lower in importance than them or are, they will offer a strong handshake. They will then entice the person physically, grab the elbow with the hand the person is shaking using an opposite hand and keep the shake for longer than usual shake.

If you are required to disarm an unforced handshake, give the handshake with a weak, limp grip. Since a broader handshake could create a feeling of discomfort, by pushing the force handshake, and then accept a lackluster limp grip in exchange, the discomfort is not the fault of the person who is pushing.

The power players can hold their appearance longer than usual alternatively creating a feeling of discomfort for the person. While the appearance isn't harmful, it's enough to cause the person look a bit uncomfortable. In response to a forceful stare is to simply walk away.

Do not fall for the tactical move and fall into an eye downward. By removing your own gaze, you provide the opportunity to reclaim your own power. They can also dictate which seat an opponent will take or by dragging out seats for you by making an inclination to sit or directing their hand toward a chair when they offer them a place. In the event you have to stop the tactic you should decide where and on how you'll be sitting before you are taken care of.

If you're gathering a group with a reputation for strategizing moves, be sure to arrive early and make sure you get the seat in first. Force players excel when it comes to making a different tend to their fellow players. If you have an organized reaching gesture, it is a sure bet that the player with force is going to make everybody look at them. Some other common characteristics of non-verbal force communication include the attack on a particular area through standing close to an alternative and touching during conversation by putting one's hands on the opposite's shoulder, or taking a hefty walking.

Ready Body Language

The body language of a confident person can trigger the excitement. Imagine a player from baseball at the outfield, ready to take on whatever ball comes in their direction. Imagine their stance, which has been prepared for non-verbal communication. A person who is ready for non-verbal communication shows the moment a person's body is in a balanced state for movement. The body's form is turned toward the direction of you are talking or the place where the movement is coming from.

Teenagers and young ladies standing her phone to get it out of her hands whenever it rings in the belief that she's waiting patiently for her lover to contact her will be primed for to communicate non-verbally. The eyes of a person will be controlled by where the event comes from. The body is agitated and ready for action, and may be playing by using their hands or twisting in a dress or a different item and awaiting movements in high vision.

The young ones display with their body language in the event that you tell them you'll be ready for departure to transport your children to the playground or the beach. However, if they're anxious about the journey like fighting, or a pupil getting prepared for the first solo exercise, they will demonstrate with a prepared non-verbal message. Brides preparing to walk through the pathway as well as Grooms looking at their partner to walk down the aisle are also displaying an organized non-verbal message.

Another example of prepared non-verbal communication that's not as obvious is where a child sits in a quiet workspace with all their equipment prepared to get started on their day. The constitution could be signalling what point the person is thinking. This could refer to an alternative one or even the entrance. The entrance could be as discrete as the foot, or as transparent as an whole form that is inclining. Eyes may also be rehashed around in the direction that is proposed. The person is anxious and ready for action. In the event of you are sitting, your hands might grip armsrests as they prepare to climb up. The legs are stretched out to move the form. The objects in the hands are kept in the hands. The hand is not considered to be a thing apart from the usual course. Hands could be able to entangle clothing, particularly with the thumbs placed into waistbands. Similar to placing hands inside pockets. It shows the individual is loos but able to be swift. When there is development and it's being planned for further development. Legs uncross. Hands snatch packs, straighten clothes, et cetera. The whole form is oriented to the typical heading.

Be Open and Relaxed

Greeting Body Language

Shaking or waving hands with someone else is a way for welcoming and greeting, however there are a variety of ways of welcoming non-verbal communications that you might not be so well-aware of. The greeting non-verbal message can be used as a cryptic signal between two people in order to show a sense of unity. A lot of groups have an unofficial handshake or hand gesture to show the commonality of their traits. Kids in elementary school frequently are the ones to have their mysterious handshakes at the club. The society that you grew up in there are a variety of non-verbal messages that you are welcome to use could not be acceptable or perhaps considered an insult.

The theory is that you could inform a crowd of people on the person's handshake. It is not a good idea without uncertainty to the individual what kind of day the individual is going through as well as a variety of other variables. The firm grip of a handshake can be a sign of the trust of the person, while a weak hand with a loose grip can be thought of as a sign of timidity. But, older ladies in particular are prone to losing their grip and may have a lightweight hand, as well as some may opt to use lighters to grip. confidence that they will make use of it to avoid having to risk having their hands crushed off!

The handshake with twofold holds with the extender shaking hands and holding their hand with the other to grip the person's elbow, or putting other hands within both of their hands is meant to display dominance. There are however a couple of individuals who when shaking hands with someone they really appreciate can include those who deliver each hand to display sincerity. Another non-verbal signal of appreciation believed to signal of power are shaking hands in a different way using the palm downwards while the palm upwards indicates submission, and the palms turned sideways indicates respect.

Handshakes that are extended to the point where one person makes it difficult for a different person to finish the salute is also sign of power. When you look attentively pictures of legislators or those in powerful post, photos of handshakes are likely to appear with people sitting shoulder-to-shoulder holding their hands and arms in front of them to accept each other's hand. The individual who has been overwhelmed is in the middle of the another person, who is shaking the left hand, and when the photo takes place, it's the second hand which is evident in the image.

There are various forms of welcoming through hand-to-hand communication. One of them is an example of the "high five" in which two people slap on the floor, clapping the hands with clenched fingers or making a gesture as the person walks past the other person in an event to acknowledge. Another form of non-verbal welcome expressions are honour, like salutes where hands are raised toward the forehead or spill of a cap, then return towards the opposite side.

The military uses salutes to display gratitude to people at higher levels. Scouts also use their own unique salute. A hand raised toward the chest when discussing how to say the Pledge of Allegiance can be a substitute of salute for honor. The bowing gesture can also be a sign of respect or indicate gratitude or gratitude, as an instance, when you are at the conclusion of an exercise. In Japan when it is observed that you do not bow during the reception, it's considered to be an indication of disrespect. respect.

Kissing and hugging are various forms of non-verbal signals, yet they ought be used with caution. A greeting to someone you do not have a relationship with by embracing them or a kiss may put you in a sour place. It is even more accepting of women embracing others in an embrace than men who embrace every one of them individually even if they are not close. Once an embrace is said more of one-sided It has gone beyond the realm of welcome and may even turn physical harassment or even striking when the person isn't an active participant.

In some society, we are relying on to thank a new acquaintance by kissing, for instance, the close kiss that is common in France and in some societies, it can be accepted as socially pleasing and it will be performed by the sex of either the other. The greeting kiss is short, like an ice cube to the lips or on the face of a different single individual. The greeting of a partner could be hugging them while watching one's cheeks or to the lips. Every kiss, of whatever length, on or off the lips, whether with closed or open mouth, is considered to be more than the sentimental touch, and is less a greeting.

It is possible to determine a person's welcoming attitude through their face expressions, too. An expression of annoyance could provide a clue of something not quite right or a stressed face and teeth that are clenched should indicate you that this person is really angry or unhappy at your actions. An expression of joy will indicate that someone is happy to have you around, whereas the appearance of a flawless face could indicate that the person might be thinking less of you or indicate that you're open to them.

When you observe an person rubbing their eyes together and rubbing their eyes, it's likely, they're trying to check your name prior to making contact with them. It's a great time to get up to them, tell them who you are, and then greet the person with a warm handshake. Some other ways to convey non-verbal welcoming include tipping your cap to show acknowledgment, and kissing your nose such as the form of an Eskimo kiss.

Chapter 4: Open Body Language

Communication that is non-verbal and open generally conveys unwinding or higher structures. Hands and arms openly convey the person's desire not to hide anything to protect themselves from an alternative. They're loose with their present situation. In the event the person is making an unspoken non-verbal message then quickly changes into an open and confident presentation this indicates a significant shift in the way they feel.

Imagine that you're speaking to a person and they're sitting position and displaying an unspoken non-verbal communication. After that, all of a suddenly they're sitting with their feet on the floor, or have risen to an upright position. You probably said something that triggered the mood to alteration. This time you can tell that your non-verbal communications may not appear as if it is displaying a loose attitude with everything, except a higher degree of fighting or unguarded non-verbal communication.

Pay attention to the words that occurred that resulted in the sudden mental state so that you can manage the conversation so that it isn't likely to trigger physical violence.

If the fingers are raised upwards the hands are held upwards, this can create an argument movement, and it could also be coupled by lowering of the body. The intention is to say 'Kindly do not hurt me'.

In supplication, opening the form also means 'Here, I can hurt you if that you would like'. It it is similar with a dog who walks across on its back, and faces the world. When there is an open body with pressure and especially when hands with clench fingers gripped, might be an indication of a significant hostility. A person is able to hold their bodies open to fight. Hostility may also be observed in the case of a form that is set onto the person next to it and generally close to the other. The changes could be unexpected and designed to check the response of another person.

The openness of a car could have a connection to a distant danger. When a person quickly 'uncovered themselves' such as by openly revealing their body and then shifting away, they're opening themselves to attack. When this happens, it could mean that they are open, they could indicate that 'I'm efficient and yet you're so weak, it is impossible to fend me off in the event that I'm visible. If the arms are positioned with palms facing each other one could be making a 'fake hug to indicate that they keep an eye on the other person. The motions could be slower, and signify elegance. There could be several motives behind the use of non-verbal communication that is open. Particularly, look for the movement in the moment that the figure is opened as well as the triggers that could be responsible for this transformation. The clothes are prone to fall around and actions that release clothing could occur like removing the coat or unbuttoning its neckline. The head could be positioned only to the person in front of it or even watching the surroundings. Eye contact could be sloppy and slow.

The legs that are open do not cross. Usually, they're straight. They can even extend to a distance. They are invested with open feet and could be indicating forward, other side, or even at an object or person or something else that's interesting. Arms aren't crossed, and can be animated and move to the beat of the words being spoken or spread wide.

The palms can also be loose, and can be very creative, as in the case of appearing to be holding objects or forming larger, more specific designs. The hands that are free show the fact that everything is not hidden.

Relaxed Body Language

Non-verbal loose communication and free non-verbal communication are a battle against with each other at loose angles. One's breathing rate is lower than usual and steady as well as overall figure influence is flexible without tension in muscles. Skin tone color is normal over the whole. The feet, hands, and arms do not seem to be nervous or shaking and lie around their laps or reclining.

Outflow of the face is loose and there's a the possibility of a slight smile or loose lips. The voice tone remains constant with the absence of overstated low or high tones. Faces will not display any scowl lines that are not properly represented. The eyes will reflect the mouth. If there is a small smile present on the lips then there's some grins on the face, and the eyebrows will be positioned in a normal manner and without effort.

The center may be sagging towards the side (not being held in place due to the occasional tension). This can also be adjustable, and the shoulders being positioned over the pelvis. It isn't likely to twist in fear, but it could twist out to a relaxed pose.breathing is constant and slower. It could cause the voice to be slightly lower than usual. The shoulders do not seem to be concerned for the majority of the time and rest in the exact position. The colour of your skin is generally normal that it isn't either reddened from shame or anger or trepidation, neither is it pale. There aren't any odd spots such as around your neck, or cheeks.relaxed Appendages are hung around. They do not wiggle and at time to time move across each other on their own, not unless it's posture of solace.

Arms that are injured can't move and are able to be closed by the body. They can move an instant or in a staccato manner. The arms that hang loosely can be inexplicably or are moved smoothly.if arms meet the arms hand around. Every intersection will be a sign of tension. The arms that are slamming down could seem comfortable.when we feel agitated often we use our hands to hold our bodies, hold us or general display strain. Hands that are loose hang off or can be used to enhance our thoughts. They're the majority of the time of the time free and can create plans that are bouncing around. The motions are fluid and gentle and not rushed or strained.

When sitting, legs may rest in a delicate position on the floor, or be tossed coolly out. They could be moved according to time to music or with tapping feet. They could be crossed however they're not wrapped over each other. The legs may be an indication of a shrouded strain whenever an individual controls the upper body and arms. If they're on a table the figure you observe may appear flexible, however legs can be tight and tucked. A person may smile softly or wildly without a hint of a grimace. The mouth generally sits still.when speaking your mouth is opened and not in a tiniest or a lot of development. The voice can sound loose, but not a surprising high volume and with no sudden shifts in speed or pitch. speed.the eyes are a bit giddy at the mouth, and especially around the tiny wrinkles on the sides of the eye.

An unintentional glance will shift towards an individual not gazing and only there is a small flash of light.

Chapter 5: Be A Gentleman

Attentive Body Language

When you're paying attention, it shows that you're listening to what other people have to have to say. Next time you talk to someone, pay particular focus on their posture as well as their eyes. The term "attentive" body language is identified as the subtle signals that you provide to someone by body language, to indicate in which you're taking note of the words that they tell you. It's normal for someone listening to mimic the body language you use. An example could be a straightforward head nod, or moving your body to be able to hear what someone else is speaking, or asking questions.

Did you stop during an exchange to ask, "Are you even listening to me?" The reason you could say this is that you noticed that the person was talking to distracted by some other thing or believed that the person wasn't listening, as evident by the numerous clues. This kind of body language is commonly referred to as an inattentive body language, which means that you are showing that you're not paying attention to the person you are talking to. As an example, you wouldn't like to hear someone else's voice whenever you are yawning during class or even in the middle of a discussion; the one exception is if you didn't get enough sleep in the previous night.

Eye contact can be an excellent way to show attention, particularly when you are attending an interview for a job. Eye contact is an essential aspect to be aware of when attending these types of job interviews. You may not believe it, but when you're focused you are less likely to blink than the average. If you're watching a good program on TV, try to notice yourself looking at the screen. There is a chance that you will see yourself, and then realize you were watching the TV while you were in the habit of paying attention to body communication.

Emotional Body Language

Non-verbal emotional communication covers an extensive area since individuals experience various distinct emotions. For instance, anger is clearly not the same thing as happy non-verbal communication. However, certain non-verbal signs that indicate joy can be triggered through tragic non-verbal messages. There are many indicators that are non-verbal and can aid in determining the way that a person is thinking about in the inner world, and regardless, they're not exclusive and all individuals respond on the identical way to the exact vibrations. Whatever you believe ought cause a person to be devastated may not actually be a factor for another.

The expression of anger can be seen within a person for a reason, ranging from receiving an unsatisfactory score on a test and a miserable working day, or missed check, to a variety of scenarios. Certain things can irritate a man much more deeply than another or faster. The most common non-verbal indicators of outrage include the flushed (red) neck or face gripped jaw or clenched hand, the pacing at a particular area or space in the other person with no regard or regard for the other, and use of forceful or combative non-verbal signals.

The feeling of tension, strain or stress can be as the same thing and are fundamental that are present in non-verbal communications. Being aware of what is happening while reading the non-verbal messages of a person will help you identify indications of improvement in your understanding of exactly which of these three emotions they're experiencing. The ability to communicate with passion can be extremely helpful in helping youngsters express the emotions that their body is experiencing. Stress, fear or stress are difficult children to discern. The fear of strain or fear non-verbally communication may be displayed in a person in their character by letting the skin with a cold sweat and a pale, dark face. mouth, and avoiding eye contact. They may appear as if you are close to tears and irritated eyes.

There could be a trembling lips or twitching eyes, vocal stammering or tremors, voices that split in the voice, sweating raised beat, held clench hands, muscles or jaw, or a broader periods of breathing. Certain individuals may appear to be agitated or agitated, while others take on their position of communication that is non-verbal. It is evident that the majority of non-verbal communications can also trigger feelings aside from fear, apprehension or anxiety. However they do so in a manner that is revealing during some time lately If you have a basic understanding of the situation it is possible to concentrate on what the individual has and how they are expressing it by their non-verbal communications before you have to connect with them.

It is helpful to determine which of the causes concern you, or if they're just worried over the situation or feeling unease about the situation. It can help you comfort your client and take a decision.

Communication that's not verbal generally manifests as a slumping of shoulders, or a figure as if it is limp an emaciated lip tears and a sluggish speech tone. The expression of embarrassment may be the appearance of a red face, an eludement or avoiding eye contact a smacked face, or an oblivious smile.

The stress of being angry can also trigger anxiety in certain people. Unexpected non-verbal communications will begin by widening the eyes and eyebrows cocked. They may open their mouths and appear to be beginning or even cause an uneasy development in the back. Non-verbal emotional communication that expresses happiness can manifest in the form of tears of joy, a smile on their eyes and mouth, as well as general discord.

A feeling of great satisfaction could be evident in someone doing what's called the joyful dance. They are jumping about. It could be that it is said or they might be falling short of with their arms or cheering with a fervent enthusiasm. While these are extremely common kinds of non-verbal communications utilized to communicate feelings people who has a certain level of influence may not display one of them. You could find them to a high degree happy and smile in the event that they choose to.

Romantic Body Language

Non-verbal emotional communication (SNS) isn't only what couples do when they're close and intimate, however even from afar. Any type of non-verbal communications can have its own book because there's a lot that can be discussed. In the case of sentimental non-verbal communication you could certainly write two books. The romantic non-verbal language combines everything from a joke to marriage, and can even cause breaking ups and divorce.

The non-verbal language of distant communication incorporates the various manifestations of what one performs with their body such as a smacking of eyelashes how they hold their bodies to the way one dress and is ready to become tease. The romantic non-verbal communications of distant origin can include sexual gestures. When you're looking to find a possible long-term real relationship, sexual gestures don't sound like a fantastic idea but in the event you are looking to add a bit of fun in the marriage of your choice, some sexually explicit non-verbal communications could provide a lot of entertainment. From a distance, the sentimental non-verbal communications can be observed in the way one presents themselves also. Women and men can dress in clothes that emphasize specific parts of their bodies that they consider attractive.

Men are known for their the non-verbal language of the pumping of specific muscles in order so that they appear larger than what they actually are. like when they position their the hands underneath their biceps in order to stretch them so that they appear bigger than what they actually are. When they meet someone who is enthralled by them then they could hold an extended flex to the final time! Females are often praised for sucking their guts to look less revealing than it really is, and then sticking their part of their midsection in order to create a bigger appearance than it really appears to be.

In the case of using emotional non-verbal communications in a distant location the individual should place themselves to appear in the eye of the investment's focus through a full turn of their either with their head or less confident person may simply turn one foot toward their preferred constantly attempting in order to make it more distinct. A person could be seen moving enticingly to the ground while watching the invest to make it is a great idea to offer an alcoholic beverage to the group of high-end.

Individual and up-close conversation should only be done if you're involved in an association with another group. If you're not engaged in a personal association with a different group it is possible to have an indexed sexual provocation claim against you. If not, it could be the worst. Communication that is intimate and non-verbal much more comfortable than communication in a distant location. The shared level of comfort allows each other to be able to step into one's own space, without others feeling shattered.

Closely-sensual non-verbal communication could show in a couple who are snarky about each other's moves, or forming poses, gazing affectionately at the eyes of each other as they sit at the television and holding hands, giving back rubs or kisses, to intimate experiences, and sexual research.

Chapter 6: Examine The Difference Between Correct Or Wrong

How am I to Identify Good from bad?

The answers below to this basic ethical question will be the basis for a book that is randomly chosen.

First, we must understand what we are referring to when we discuss morality and right to understand the moral nuances that we need to develop. It is my goal to develop G.E. Moore's moral perspective that is not naturalistic that he formulated in the perspective of his Principia Ethica (1903). According to Moore's perspective, morality could be viewed as a type of universal quality. Within this moral spectrum that ranges from extremely positive to incredibly evil, as well as neutral to the middle, all actions have a place.

I'd like to compare morality with time in the present. It is impossible to point out any specific feature in the world.

The same is true for morality, too. If we are witness to a crime and claim that it's wrong and we don't point to an actual physical object of "wrongness but instead highlight a virtue that's inherent to the incident. The moral aspect can be seen so that we are able to perceive moral qualities.

You might wonder if one can comprehend moral fact such a way that there's still an overwhelming debate on moral questions. Moral facts don't have to be so simple, such as 'killing people is wrong' or 'being useful is good. The act of killing isn't wrong because someone might just murder someone to stop the explosives from detonating in a classroom.

The actions of an individual can have diverse motives as well as unknown details. In order to determine if something complicated is ethical, it is necessary to understand not just what we are doing, but also the motive as well as the motivation of the person who took an action and its expected effect. Moral wisdom can be obtained by analyzing the perceptions that a person gets about an act and analyzing the thoughts of the individual that took the decision.

Certain people are more adept in understanding these perceptions, and transforming these into information. It's not to make ethicists into a priesthood of morality. The way to think of it is, as my metaethics professor stated as akin to space. Someone might constantly smack their head because of a absence of spatial awareness. All of us can gain greater comprehension of morality by becoming more aware of our moral perceptions.

There's no formula that works however there's a way which can help you in times where there is doubt. To begin, you must determine what the circumstances are. Uncertainty never makes for good decision-making. Allow others to impose upon the facts you'd rather not consider.

In the second and most challenging part attempt to anticipate the results of choices you may make. Even the most well-planned results can result in unimaginable effects. Even the most committed person who is not concerned about consequences must take into account the fact that giving others benefits is a fundamental moral concept, even if it's is not a guiding one.

Thirdly, consider the moral tenets which force that you should do something or another. These principles should be pertinent and valid, something that can be argued. Catholics believe that divorce is incorrect, but Islam facilitates divorce for both men and women. It is your belief that we should be respectful of the sacredness of the life of a murderer; I believe that the concept that life is sacred has been discarded by the murderers. Then, make the choice.

Unfortunately, the validity and relevance of moral standards clash and it is possible to choose which ought to follow from two relevant arguments. My view believes that the primary aim is often the one that will bring maximum good into the world. But it is not necessarily the case.

There is a higher duty towards some people than others and this is in conflict with my obligation to save more lives than those less fortunate. However, I'll protect my child more than the ten other strangers. Morality was born out of the concern for family members and it is important not to wander too far from the deepest roots.

Furthermore, some values may be more fundamental over other ones. It might be more crucial not to sacrifice an innocent life rather than help save it. Therefore, I shouldn't take one life to save another. What if I could make fifty lives better by killing only one?

Morality may be contingent on situations, but not absolute but at some point the utilitarian concept prevails. Examining similar situations in which it is obvious that the solution is beneficial; observing the ways they differ from present situation helps to clarify thinking. Also, always talk about issues with the people you trust as well as those who don't agree with your views. If you do something wrong apologize, then strive to improve next time.

The best approach to address this issue is to look at commonly-held ethics and examine these for the particular situation in hand. This is because adhering to an ethical principle that generally, it is a solid base for ethical actions. A good example of this could be one of them is the Golden Rule ('do unto others in the same way as you'd want them to do to you) which is found in a myriad of faith and religion practices.

It is believed that concepts like this provide reliable evidence of 'rights or wrongs' can be compelling. Moralists have argued that ethical behavior is rooted in a sense of duty and it is not a result of innate genetic predisposition towards good behavior. Being aware of the responsibilities that others have rather than self-interest can appear morally beneficial.

Additionally, in line with Kant theorists, there are those who believe that we should not view others simply as means to attain a desired goal, but as an end in itself in their own right', recognizing their ability for moral thought. The idea of treating people as the goal, and not as a method, is ethical as it's compassionate and considerate of other people; one of the essential qualities to ethics-based behavior.

The strict application of ethical guidelines could have apparent ethical implications. A majority of people think it is wrong to tell the truth in almost all circumstances but it is acceptable to be honest in certain situations like in order to save the life of a person.

In addition, a strong emphasis on duty's importance could give the impression that ethics are a complex and difficult concept but this isn't entirely persuasive: it is hard to accuse the naturally generous individual as not being ethical since they don't do so in a spirit of obligation.

In the end, while most of us believe that we ought to appreciate and respect other people however, we might be willing to treat people as a way to achieve it is likely to yield significantly better outcomes. As an example, lots of people believe that it's appropriate to risk the life of a single person to save a number of lives. It is also wrong to sacrifice a life. This is why, even though there are many who have clear opinions that tell them what is correct or unjust however, they do recognize the fact that sometimes adhering to rigidly the same rules is unwise and unethical which makes ethics as uneasy just like other branches of the humanities.

It means that moral judgements regarding right and wrong are challenging, and crucial ethical issues remain unanswered.

Philosophers may debate many various theories, but ultimately I'd suggest an easy boo-hoo approach in separating correct from incorrect. It's okay, I'm not looking for psychopaths.

However, I believe that most people have a deep displeasure at morally indecent behaviors that stem from compassion. If you're trying to determine what actions you take towards an person are morally correct or not you can ask yourself whether that's the way you'd like to treat them. This is the objectiveity that we are living, conscious beings. What's more complicated than the fact that we're aware?

This could be from this question that the process of determining the right from the wrong is fundamentally cognitive. Therefore, employing the language of Benjamin Bloom's Taxonomy of learning objectives within the cognitive realm I'm able to remember things considered to be wrong or right and understand the reasons for why they're such. I am able to apply my memory and knowledge of what is correct and incorrect to make decisions appropriate in certain situations and analyze the actions and identify which are correct and which are not; I determine if something is correct or not I am able to formulate precise and nuanced concepts of the rightness or wrongness. The knowledge I acquire is gained through experimentation and derived from the responses from other people's reactions in response to my actions or say.

It is, however, an important issue as the responses of others in my statements or words cause me to feel emotions. In order to use Bloom for this purpose first, I pay attention to specific activities that evoke reactions from other people or emotions in my. I develop the ability to be responsive to certain actions under specific situations by other people. It is also my experience that certain responses are appreciated by other people or me. I arrange some of the appreciated responses using certain guidelines.

In the end, these concepts interconnect and my behavior is defined by these principles.

Because right and wrong do not exist apart from the conscious of all the world's people at any given moment It is feasible to make a decision on the basis of retrospect. It is possible to argue that shifting beliefs are a sign of inherent wrongness with regards to specific actions, maybe leading to an inherent order of good and evil like discovering the physical laws.

However, these beliefs have proven not to be true before. Since the beginning of time, people believed that the Bible provided certain answers. However, If a creator were to come out and declare that "Same-sex marriage is not right" or 'Capital Punishment is the right thing to do', lots of people, like myself, would be in difficulties accepting this. We'd instantly know what is right and what isn't, but believe that a lot of 'right' items were wrong as well.

A few elements of the what is right and wrong might seem obvious however, for the major of the time, we need to be guided by our morals. This is why there is no guarantee. All I can do is try my best.

The simple answer is that I am unable to. Professor. Oliver Scott Curry of Oxford University has essentially cracked the morality puzzle, using empirical data of sixty different cultures, both present as well as historical. This is my version on his initial thoughts which is why the book you've been reading ought to be given to the author.

As with Rome with its hills morality is based on the seven natural values that are held in varying degree, with the purpose of encouraging cooperation and resolving conflicts. Most important among them are Possession which is regarded as sacred by 9-tenths of the cultures as well as the laws. Following are loyalty, Kinship and reciprocity, which are believed to be a virtue by a quarter of the population. Nearly half of all cultures value the importance of respect (for the strong) as well as Humility (of the weak). The last and most important is Fairness which is valued only by 15 percent. Dosvidanya socialism is another example, but do not give a crook an opportunity to even. Everyone has the right to claim his own unique principle, as well as aesthetics and aesthetics, but only seven values are truly common.

Societies and cultures differ on the extent and importance they place on these seven moral pillars. The right thing to do is help attain a conscious or subconscious purpose, such as reproducibility, social cohesion longevity, wealth, or even conquest. The wrong is the thing that hinders the aim, while wrong is seen as being done this intentionally.

Different values may conflict and one can be a detriment to another, resulting in disastrous consequences. If the aim is to exercise absolute dominance over submission to absolute authority, for ever?

What are we able to say regarding this question? We must first have the answer. We are already aware of what the terms 'right' and wrong' means. If we did not, we'd be confused by the topic. Yet, at the time there are disagreements with other people on what is right as well as wrong. If we can tell the difference between the right way and wrong way the only thing we must be able to do is clarify what these terms mean when we speak of them. Then, the other will be able to explain what they're talking about, and then our evident disagreements will be settled?

But we can't do that. It is possible to examine an act, agree completely on the facts, regarding the substance of the action and the effects it will have, but differ on whether the action is correct. If this is true, then you should not be debating the essence of what we are discussing. We disagree - and the meaning we all have of "right" must be in another place.

This is the reason there are times when we cannot agree on the correctness of an action. the degree to which it is right is only a matter of comparison with other actions.

Which actions then? If we could identify the characteristic that differentiates 'right actions' from those that aren't and defined what we were referring to when we spoke of rightness and wrongness. However, if we did the same, we'd return to the right and wrongness in relation to a truth, and all apparent differences would turn out to be just misunderstandings.

Our inability to reach a consensus suggests that this can't be true. If both right and wrong are the graduations of the same system, and if it is the case that we can't define boundaries to this system, then that system is bound to include all things. Which kinds of systems have all things, or attempt to? They are philosophical in nature. Therefore, I believe that our perception of what is the right and wrong are determined by the way we think. As long as there is a common philosophical framework, we already have a clear idea of what is what is right and incorrect. If we're not sure of these, it's because the philosophy we have isn't formed inside our heads.

What is the reason we should be able of discerning what is right and what isn't? Morality doesn't exist in our universe in the way the laws are portrayed by nature and is a matter of choice for humans, and individuals choose to react to moral dilemmas in a variety of manners.

The utilitarian systems of Bentham and Kant's deontology offer crucial insights. However, they each have their own drawbacks, the one for its blatant indifference to innocent people's (assumed) rights, and the second is its inability to consider implications. But what's the basis that we use to evaluate the obvious flaws in both of these systems? According to positivists it's all about psychology that is based on evolution as well as upbringing.

Do these results lead to relativism which is a contradiction in of not intervening in another's society or critique the psychopath? No, I'm not sure. In most societies, the notion of inflicting pain and suffering on innocent people is a slap in the face. Because of a gut instinct or psychological inclination We know (or are we convinced?) that this type of violence is unjust.

If we adhere to certain guidelines, our society will provide us with outcomes that coincide with our moral beliefs. In many societies, individuals share these ideals to provide an impression of a common goal to pursue ethical behavior. What's the reason we shouldn't try to convince other people that we live a lifestyle of living that is compatible with our psychological needs as well as ours?

Chapter 7: Understanding Why People Lie

In the current world that which we live in the present, lying is a reality that occurs, not unlike groups which specialize in debunking truths often shared in public declarations and press releases that currently exist.

Naturally, not just businessmen and politicians be lying to us. It doesn't matter if it's the child sitting in front of the broken vase which says he didn't break or the teenager who gives reasons for why she went to bed over two hours after her bedtime the night before, lies are common throughout the homes of most families.

The reasons behind many lies are not clear. Sometimes, the purpose is to protect a liar from punishment, or shield others from

punished or exempt someone else from being punished. Its purpose might be to hide embarrassing circumstances, keep from embarrassment, or to make another person feel good in their own self-esteem. Even though lying in public is not acceptable, it's not difficult to understand why it occurs.

It's even hard to grasp the reasons why certain people regularly make up stories that serve an undefined purpose, but generally are easy to disprove.

According to studies that have conducted research, there is a myriad of reasons that can be attributed to certain individuals' habitual lying.

Another is that the person lying may be unaware that it's an untruth. Repeated liars can experience severe tension to the point where their memory becomes impaired. When they say anything to assist in completing the situation the liars attempt to ease the stress.

Doesn't feel comfortable with this type of command, they come up with an untruth that is in fact conforms to their desired narrative.

They may be worried that if they tell the truth, it will make their appearance look unflattering and they'll be criticized. Instead, they create some falsehood to make themselves appear attractive, however they don't always realize the fact that their statements aren't grounded in reality.

It would be wonderful to believe everything we heard, no matter if it was from a small child who held the broken vase, or from a politician at a gathering. However, since this isn't likely be the case, it's vital for us all to sometimes dig further and find the facts.

We don't all wish to be constantly told the facts. Imagine someone asking whether you look like a woman. This is the problem that arises in situations where people justify the usage of "nonwhite" falsehoods as essential and justifiable. It is common for relationships to be destroyed once an untruth is discovered.

The consequences of lying can be devastating. The perceptions of someone else about you can change when they find out about your lying. There is a possibility that you can resolve your problems with your spouse's lying during the counseling room, however an employer will not accept your explanation.

We often do not want to be around people who are lying, however truthfully, all of us have a tendency to lie at time to time. They come in all shapes and styles, from exaggeration of facts to complete fake news. It's not unreasonable to conclude that lying is innate since many children are lying without even realizing it.

However common lying is yet, it's still considered unprofessional and a bad act. The act of being lied to is difficult and often violates the bonds of trust between two individuals, which can cause difficulties in the relationship. Understanding the motives behind why lies are committed could shed clarity on the situation and assist us in understanding the individuals who commit a lie. Let's an examination of some typical reasons people are lying.

Self-Defense

Most individuals lie in order to shield themselves from unfavorable situations or conflicts. Consider the young kids who tell lies; they are doing it in order to ensure that they won't be in troubles. Kids lie to avoid adversity penalties or consequences. Adults are the same way. A lot of people lie when they're aware that they've committed a crime which could cause anger to others.

The woman could cover up the expense of her shoes while a man could make up a story about who that he would meet up with.

The truth is that they are used for protection from punishment or to keep a peace. It is possible that the person has not committed any wrongdoing, but like to not be forced the need to justify their actions, defend themselves or deal with an angry spouse. To Spare Feelings

A few people who lie frequently have intention to do so with good motives. They are referred to as "white lies" which are committed when a person is trying to prevent causing another hurt. An erroneous husband could lie to protect his wife's feelings and a father might be lying to prevent his kid from experiencing crying. An example of a typical white lie is "Yes Dear, that gown looks gorgeous for you."

For some, the white lie may be nothing more than an argument or excuse, rather than an falsehood. The ethics behind the telling of the truth is a subject of debate all in the past by philosophers and theologians. Every person must determine whether telling a lie is acceptable. If preventing someone from getting wounded in the process means that they are not telling all truth and nothing result from the falsehood the majority of people will believe that the act is not just acceptable but are also convinced that it is.

To safeguard feelings individuals who lie are trying to shield their feelings and avoid causing someone else suffering or harm, the majority of are lying to safeguard their self-esteem, feelings, confidence in their own self, or another private feelings. Someone who claims, "I didn't want that job in the first place," when she did lie to defend her feelings. If a child yells, "I hate you!" could be trying to shield his self from being hurt, or even to avoid being rejected by others prior to they are disapproved of.

To Keep a Secret

If one is thinking about fabrications of lies in order to hide something from the public One must be thinking of Christmas or birthdays. A lot of people cover up their whereabouts or the things they purchased in the hope to keep a sense of excitement. The majority of time they appear to be obvious. The teen may have a clue she was taken out by her mom however something about her mother's reason for leaving raises suspicion.

If the truth is revealed and a teenager gets a lovely present for an occasion The lie is then forgiven and put to rest.

to present a good image People want to create the best image possible, usually because of work reasons. Consider an interview in which an individual might wear a nice outfit and make an effort to impress the person interviewing them in order to get the job. The people who lie to hide their reasons of appearance usually do it as a way of glossing over an issue on their resume or refrain from supplying the true reasons for the termination at a previous employer.

To Be Liked

Everybody wants to be liked and to be part of a group is essential and is a the human condition. People lie in order to get the attention of other people. Someone may pretend to have an interest in a subject or even agree with something that they is not sure about. The issue that could arise when a person is caught in this kind of deceit is the lack of personal identity in addition to being incapable of being yourself. To Manipulate Others

It is quickly learned that we are able to manipulate the behavior of others. If we decide to manipulate others is an issue of discussion.

It is a fact that a lot of individuals lie in order to convince the other person to do the things they would like they want them to do. The people who use lies to influence the situation or to manipulate other people usually only care about the gain of their own and don't think about the opinions of other people. Through lying or not mentioning details they can accomplish an individual goal.

But, it's important to remember that lying can alter a circumstance and individual's thinking; it's not just lying without intention. The way we talk and act impacts others. Even well-intentioned lies can be a method of manipulating. A Matter of Trust

The act of lying can create a stressful situation as we believe that people behave with respect and to tell the truth. We do not want to be deceived by others or manipulated. When the incident occurs that we are lied to, we have lost confidence and faith on the person we are dealing with. Some individuals (typically people with particular personality issues) who are known to lie often and don't care about the results they cause by their lying. These types of people usually does not take into consideration how he is treated by others.

However, most people are concerned about how other people are treated, and knowing that they have been lied to could cause a breach in trust, contingent on the severity of the deceit. How we view things affects our perception of lies and the consequences that lie can bring about in itself. Many people think that politicians are lying. As it's normal, it is accepted.

This is also true for used car salespersons. Very few people feel the loss of trust when people are lying and continue to live their lives without causing any repercussions.

Compulsive and Pathological Lying

An even more severe issue that lies can cause is when it turns into a pathological or compulsive habit. There are differences between these two aren't obvious, but it's crucial to know the difference between them. The compulsive lier uses lying as a method of living. The act of lying in any circumstance or at any time is a substitute for honesty.

An obsessive liar is one who lies since it benefits the individual in a strange way, and they take comfort by lying. Truth isn't right for someone who has a tendency to modify the truth in order to meet his own desires and needs. It is usually coupled with issues with personality such as Narcissism. Although the person engaging in the habit feels safe however, they can hurt and harm relationships, families as well as family members. The habit of lying can be addictive and is hard to kick after it becomes habitual.

The pathological liar is constantly lying to obtain what they want with no regard for anyone those who are hurt on the route. As a way to cope for pathological lying, these people often have various personality issues.

The words that define a pathological liar include deceitful as well as manipulative and self-centered. The pathological liar will tell the truth and may even alter their story between telling and telling. Some people are aware of the lies however the lying liar usually doesn't and shows no regrets.

It is common for her to make up stories as she goes and will rarely plan an elaborate lie. When confronted, she'll justify the lie but will often deny that she has was lying. The lies told by a pathological lie can be absurd, for instance, she claims that you were at the park watching people and observed the perpetrator of a crime, but actually she was out shopping with a companion. Being a victim of a compulsive, or pathological liar can be enough to test patience with loved ones. It is a habit and pathological lies are an identity disorder.

How to Tell if Someone Is Lying

A person who tells a lie frequently will give clues that the information being stated is not real. It could be through the body language, facial expressions and even the words someone is saying. A person who is telling lies typically sweats, or appears anxious and nervous. The absence of eye contact or eyes that wander while telling a story top the list of indicators to recognize if someone's lying. People who lie will speak by raising the tone that they speak.

Your body language can tell a story of deceit. The most common method used by liars is to place something like an article, book or notebook, in front of their body to deceive others.

In this way by lying, the person who lies creates herself in a way that is unwelcome to another person. The lie-teller may distance herself from you, either by turning her back or making a move away. The gestures that are pronounced in the act of telling a lie begin by gently rubbing the forehead, kissing lips frequently, swallowing difficult, and then wringing your hands. Instead of smiling naturally an eloquent person will insist on to smile with the mouth as if it is smiling however, not with eyes. If you ask an inquiry such as "Did you get money from my wallet?" The liar is likely to reply to the question with "I didn't take the money out of your purse." They will then ask the same query to you again and not use the phrase "didn't."

Other signs that lie is being revealed include giving excessive information and monotone voice. The longer the lie-teller talks, and the longer they talk, the higher the chance that that the truth will be revealed and you must offer the person enough rope to hang him.

Being able to tell if the person you are talking to is lying is usually impossible, and the only method of determining the truth is to make an admission. If you are the next time you suspect that someone may be lying to you be aware of the body language and facial expressions for signs that the indicators of the lies are apparent. There's no way to tell whether they are lying yet, but it's an interesting thing to test. Though this list may not be complete, it gives an intriguing look at the causes of lying, and can help ease an uncomfortable circumstance.

If you discover that your spouse lies about his location, and not due to the lie is a ploy to cheat against you, but because he is afraid to be a target because he's been late and this will give you security. If you believe that your child is lying due to the fact that she's feeling limited by the rules you set it is possible to discuss granting the teen more freedom, and you are likely to receive more respect.

Chapter 8: How To Recognize The Signs That Someone Is Lying

Tips for Identifying Lying

The act of lying and deceit is a normal human behavior. Up until recently it was difficult to conduct real-world research on how frequently individuals lie. An 2004 Reader's Digest poll found that nearly 96% of respondents acknowledge that they lie at least sometimes.1

The study, which was published nationally in 2009, surveyed 1000 U.S. adults and found that 60% of the respondents declared that they did not tell the truth at all. However, they discovered that around 50% of lies were being told by five percent of thesubjects.2The research suggests that although there are a variety of rates but there is some very notorious lie-tellers.

In reality, most people be lying every time from time to time. Many of the lies we hear are harmless white lies designed to safeguard others' feelings ("No this shirt will not look fat! !").

However, in other instances, these are more dangerous (like using a fake resume) or more sinister (covering the truth of a crime).

It is surprising how poorly people are in detecting lying. A study, for instance discovered that participants had the ability to discern lying 54 percent in the majority of time in a laboratory environment. That's not amazing when considering an average detection rate of 50% just by luck alone.3

It is evident that differences in the behavior of honest and lying people are very difficult to discern and evaluate. Researchers have been trying to find several ways of detaching the lies.

There may not be any obvious and definite indication that someone is lying (like pinocchio's nose) However, research has found some useful indicators.

As with many other things it is true that spotting a lie usually boils down to trusting your intuition. Knowing the indicators that can be a reliable indicator of a lie, as well as learning to listen to your instincts and feelings, you could be able improve your ability to spot the lies.

Press Play for Advice On Lying

The show is hosted by editor-in-chief and therapist Amy Morin, LCSW, this episode of The Verywell Mind Podcast, with psychotherapist Paul Ekman aka "the human lie detector" explains why people lie, and how you can discern whether the person you're talking to is lying. You can listen to the episode below.

Signs of Lying

Psychologists have conducted research into the body language and deceit in order to aid police distinguish between real and the false. Researchers from UCLA did research regarding the topic and also analyzed sixty studies about deception in an effort to develop suggestions and guidelines for law enforcement personnel. Their findings have been released in the journal American Journal of Forensic Psychiatry.4

The Signs of a Person Who Could Have Been Lying Among possible red flags researchers discovered that may suggest that someone is deceiving could be:

The answer is vague, with only a some details, but not responding

Inability to provide precise information whenever a story has been called into question

Hair grooming activities like using hair to play with or pressing fingers on lips. The lead researcher R. Edward Geiselman suggests that even though recognizing deceit can be difficult, high-quality training may improve someone's capability to recognize lies:

"Without the right training, many believe that they are able to spot deceit However, their perceptions do not correspond to the actual capabilities. Inexperienced, short-term training can lead to think too much and perform better than if they just go by their instincts. "4

Tips for Identifying Lying

If you believe that you are not in fact telling the truth There are some methods you could employ to help you distinguish truth from fiction.

In identifying the lies of others, we tend to look at the body communication "tells," or subtle signals that are physical or behavioral that indicate deceit. Though body language clues may be a clue to deceit but research indicates that certain behaviors expected do not necessarily indicate being lying.

One of the most reliable tricks that people look out for are:

Unclarity The speaker appears to deliberately leave out crucial information, it could be because they're lying.

Uncertainty in the voice: If a person appears unsure or uneasy and uncertain, they're most likely seen as being deceitful.

Lack of interest: A lack of expression or an uninterested posture could be indicators of lying as they are all trying to keep from expressing feelings and possibly telling.

Thinking too much: If the person appears to be thinking way too much in order to understand all the details this could mean that they're deceiving you.

This is a lesson that even though body language can assist, it's essential to focus on specific signals. But, there are some who suggest that too much reliance on particular signals can hinder the ability to spot lies.

Ask Them to Tell Their Story in Reverse

Lie detection may be viewed as an inactive process. Many people believe that they are able to simply observe a potential lie-teller's facial expressions and body language in order to identify evident "tells." When you adopt a the initiative in finding out lies, you will get more effective outcomes.

A few studies have suggested the idea that having people report their experiences in reverse rather than chronological order may improve the effectiveness of detecting lies. Non-verbal and verbal signals which distinguish between lies and telling the truth could become obvious as we increase our cognitive load.

It is mentally more taxing than being honest. If you are adding more cognitive complexity, the behavioral signals might become clearer.

In addition, lying more cognitively challenging, but those who lie spend more energy to monitor their behavior and the reactions of other people. They're concerned about their credibility, and making sure that they are believed by others. It takes a large amount of time, and it is a good idea to add an extremely difficult job (like the telling of the story backwards) Cracks in the narrative and various behavior indicators could be easier to detect.

In one research, more than 80 suspects who were mocked were either truthful or made up stories about a fake incident. The participants were required to tell their experiences in reverse order, while other people simply reported their experiences in chronological sequence. The study found that reverse-order interviews provided greater behavioral evidence of deceit.

As part of a follow-up experiment, 55 police officers were shown video recordings from the previous study and were asked identify the truth and who did not.

The inquiry found that law enforcement officials could detect more falsehoods in reverse-order interviews as opposed to chronological interviews.10

Trust Your Instincts

The immediate reactions of your gut may be more precise than any lying detection that you may attempt. In a study, researchers were able to have 72 participants view videos of mock interviews with crime suspects.11Some of the suspects obtained a $100 cash note on a bookcase, whereas others were not. However, they were all instructed to inform the interviewer they didn't have any cash.

As with previous studies however, the subjects were unable to discern lies consistently and only correctly identifying lying people 40 percent in the time and truth-tellers 48% time.11

Researchers also employed implicit behavioral reactions time tests to measure their participants' more conscious and automatic responses to subjects.

They found that subjects were more likely to subconsciously connect words such as "dishonest" as well as "deceitful" to the people who were actuallylying.11 Also, they were more likely to subconsciously associate terms like "valid" as well as "honest" with truth-tellers.

These results indicate that individuals could have an intuition about when they are lying.

In other words, if our intuitions may be more precise Why aren't we more adept at detecting dishonesty? The conscious response could interfere with our instinctual associations. Instead of basing ourselves on our intuitions, we focus on the stereotyped behaviors people often identify with lying, like the tendency to fidget and a lack of eye contact.7 Insisting on behavior that does not reliably indicate deceit, makes it difficult to differentiate between reality and fiction.

A Word From Verywell

It is true that there isn't a universal, certainfire indicator of lying. Every one of the indicators of behavior, signs, and indications that have been linked by researchers to lying are just indicators that can help determine if the person in question is truthful.

The next time you're trying to assess the credibility of a story told by someone else look beyond the familiar "lying indicators" and discover how to recognize more subtle actions which could be a sign of the deceit. If necessary, adopt an active role by putting pressure on the person and making lying harder on the mind by having the individual tell the story in reverse the order.

And, perhaps the most important, trust your gut. It is possible that you have an instinctive sense of honesty versus fraud. Take note of your gut emotions.

Chapter 9: Strategies For Determining The Truth

How do you know if you are being deceived? The ability of a person to detect the lie is just higher than figuring out the flip of the coin. However, it's more easy to discern if someone is lying if they're covered in the veil, says new research.

The idea was conceived by scientists from The University of Ontario Institute of Technology in Canada and at the University of Amsterdam in the Netherlands. They recorded two video clips of a woman observing the bag of a stranger, one of which featured the woman taking items from the bag. Then, they played either one as well as the second video to female witnesses who were designated for the role of "witnesses". Following this, witnesses were required to "testify" before the camera that they did not witness the woman take anything

The result was that half of the participants actually told the truth, while half were forced to be lying. The participants were all driven by the prize of $50 if they convinced others that they were true.

The veil of Truth

After the researchers showed these videos to the other participants, they discovered that they had a much higher accuracy in determining whether the woman was lying or not when they were wearing the hijab or niqab.

The reason could be that when it was that way, the audience was less likely to judge based on the appearance. When it comes to the the veil might have focused the attention of the eyes of women, helping to keep out distractions. People who were lying made little eye contact with camera than those who could be found telling the truth. Hence, paying attention to the eyes of people who wear niqabs may help others recognize the difference.

The same study suggests that niqabs led the participants wearers to share more information verbally than those who were wearing hijabs or a veil. The veil provided more data on which the viewers could make their judgements based on changing the emphasis off of body and appearance communication.

This discovery is fascinating considering an incident in 2013 UK legal case where an judge directed the defendant accused of harassing a witness to strip her veil. Judge argued that it was essential to look her in the face in order to determine how honest she really was - however, these findings suggest it was not an appropriate decision.

Although the lying spotters were more precise for women who were covered in a veil, they nevertheless showed some predisposition. This could be because of their desire to prove they were not prejudiced. If women wore a hijab put on, they could be more inclined to believe that she had told the truth.

The function of eyes in detecting lies is complex. It is widely believed that "liars gaze upwards as well as towards the left" however this theory is now disproved as there's no link between lying and the direction your eyes are moving in. The frequency of blinks doesn't appear to correlate with the telling of lies either. Eye contact as well as speech patterns appear to be the most reliable ways to spot a fake by observation.

Our odds of detaching lies from approximately 50:50 remains identical when reading papers as well. A team headed by Stephan Ludwig at the University of Westminster, UK, has recently experimented with computer-generated text analysis which produced astonishing outcomes.

Researchers developed a model which looks for clues in a language which could signal a lie such as the absence of personal pronouns, such as "I" as well as "you" that could suggest that someone is trying to disengage themselves from the words they're using.

Additionally, they made the model evaluate factors like an attitude of self-pity or flattery.

For testing to test it, they worked in partnership with a tech company which is often required to spot fraudulent business communications. The trial involved the model was able to analyze over 8000 emails that bid for prizes based on the firm's efficiency. Utilizing text mining software, the model analysed the bids to win fibs which was then evaluated against the results of an independent audit conducted by the Account managers at the company.

The examination confirmed that the algorithm correctly classified 70 percent of reward request as deceptive or truthful. Anyone who reads those emails could have more harm.

Machine prosecutors

It is important to keep in mind that we've tried using technology to spot lies in the past and failed. Methods like the polygraph test have been generally viewed as a pseudoscience. However, they are not stopping from being used by police departments throughout the UK and across the world. Every human has the capacity to lie. We all do numerous research has shown that in the average Americans are prone to telling at least two or three lies per every day. However, experts suggest that there is a way to recognize the signs of lying.

In order to identify a fraud, first you must be aware of the way someone behaves in the event of honesty, according to Traci Brown, a body expert in language and the author of How to Spot Lies, Fraud and Identity Theft Field Guide. Watch, for instance, the way someone answers an unassuming question like, "Where are you from?" Where do their eyes turn? What is their voice like?

After you've determined the foundation, watch for changes in the behavior of four distinct categories: body language and facial expressions, as well as tone of voice, as well as the contents of speech, according to the psychologist Dr. Lillian Glass, author of The Body Language of

Liars. "Those are the rules of communications," she says.

However, the signs don't guarantee anything for instance, if someone feels unhappy in their seats it's possible they'll fidget. If someone is anxious or anxious, their voice could be shaky.

"There are debates within the medical community, especially on the subject of mental health, on which indicators of body language that could be used to determine if the person is lying." claims the Dr. Gary Brown, a licensed marriage and family Therapist based out of Los Angeles.

Our mental perceptions could hinder our ability to read the signals, says doctor. Jenny Taitz, a Clinical psychologist based in Los Angeles. "It isn't easy to interpret the signals of someone's body language accurately. the body language of a person because they might appear tense or uncomfortable for a variety of motives," she says. "For instance, it's not difficult to envision avoiding eye contact, something that is often associated with lying and for a variety of reasons ranging from being uncomfortable or a bit bored, or embarrassed because you realize that you're being deceitful. There are times when we're not as skilled at recognizing others' actions than we believe."

There are certain signals that experts recommend being on the lookout for.

Body Cues

Hands: Lies often make gestures with their hands following a conversation instead of during or prior to a conversation according to Traci Brown. Brown has taken part in a deceit training program that was run by people from the FBI and has occasionally assisted on investigation. "The mind can be doing various things like making up the truth, trying to determine the truth, and then adding details to the story in the process," she says. "So it's a common gesture that is usually made just prior to making a statement occurs following the fact."

A study from 2015 conducted at the University of Michigan looked at 120 clips from courts with high stakes to learn the way people act when they lie and when they're honest. It was found that people lying people are more likely to use their hands simultaneously when they're honest The participants yelled both hands in 40 percent of lying videos as opposed to 25% of honest clips.

If people are untruthful, they tend to keep their hands away from you, suggests Traci Brown. She regularly delivers keynote talks for financial institutions in order to assist identify and avoid fraud. This is a subconscious signal they are avoiding facts, emotions or lying, she explains. "They might place them in pockets or slip them underneath the table."

Fidgeting and itching: swaying your body around or cocking the head towards the side, or moving feet are also indications of fraud, claims Glass who has was awarded a postdoctoral position at UCLA with a focus on Psychology as well as Verbal as well as Non-Verbal Communication.

The autonomic nervous system, which controls body functions, could affect the body on the body, says. In the event of nervousness and experiencing stress, the fluctuations of the nervous system may cause individuals to experience itching or sensations of tingling in their bodies that in turn trigger more sweating as she describes.

Studies done by UCLA psychologist R. Edward Geiselman drew an identical conclusion. They found that most people exhibit "grooming behavior," such as playing with their hair while being untruthful.

Facial Cues

Eyes: A person who is lying could look or look away for an important moment, according to Glass -- which could be a indication that they're looking around while trying to figure out what they should think of the next time.

The study carried out by Geiselman at UCLA found this to be true, revealing that some people turn their eyes away when they lie. A study from 2015 conducted by University of Michigan also found that people who lie had a higher likelihood of looking at in the direction of those who had been honest -- to the point that 70 percent of videos of those who were lying had they were looking directly at individuals they had been lying to.

There's still a debate about this issue, but. The study from 2012 released in Plos One disproved the notion that people stare towards a particular direction when they're dishonest. There is the possibility that you read too much into a person's habits, Glass maintains that there can be some truth that could be been gleaned from eyes.

A mouth that rolls your lips to an extent that they nearly disappear may be a sign one is lying through or omission, says Traci Brown. "It's my personal experience that when people do this, they're denying feelings or even facts," she says.

The research conducted by UCLA revealed that people who lie more likely to follow their lips when they are asked difficult questions. The lips' pursuit could suggest that someone isn't ready to participate in the discussion in front of them, according to Glass. "It's a reflex that's instinctual, meaning that you're not going to talk," she says.

A change in appearance: Have you ever noticed someone appear as white as ghostly when they speak? This could be an indication of lying, according to Glass who believes that this indicates blood flowing out of the facial area.

Dryness, or sweating Changes in the autonomic nervous system may cause people to sweat around the T-zone on the facial area (upper lips, forehead, the chin and the area around the mouth) or suffer from dryness of the mouth and around their eyespeople may over blink or squint, chew or bite their lips, or take a big swallow, according to Glass.

Find the most up-to-date career health, relationship and wellness information to enhance your life Join Time's Living Newsletter.

Tone of Voice

High-pitched voices: If you're stressed out and stressed, muscles around the vocal cords could get tighter (an natural tension response) which causes your voice to sound high pitched, according to Glass. There could also be an itch in the voice of someone else.

The throat is cleared, which is to ease the pain of tight muscles, could occasionally signal disloyalty the doctor says.

An abrupt change in volume. People who fb are also known to increase their voice, according to Glass. "Sometimes it's because you'll become angry," she adds.

Content of Speech

Expressions like 'I'd like to be truthful with you', 'honestly and honestly' or 'I'll be honest with you are signs you're trying too hard to impress you with their truthfulness, according to Glass.

Making use of words like "uh," "like" or 'um'. research carried out at the University of Michigan found "speaking by using more vocal fill" is a typical indication of deceit. Glass states that people tend to make use of these terms often when trying to purchase time to determine what they'll say in the future.

We slip-up: The majority of us aren't natural lie-tellers, Glass notes. We can let the truth get out. See someone saying, "I was fired -I'm sorry and I'm not saying that I have quit" or "I had dinner out with So and So -- but in reality it was because I worked at night." There's a chance you're some liars on your hands She claims.

Chapter 10: Secrets Of Lie Detecting

(BODY LANGUAGE)

There is a chance that you have heard from Koko the gorilla. She was a signer. Koko was also known for her cat, All Ball. A few days ago, Koko was getting naughty, and took her sink off from the wall. As her caretakers asked her about it, she informed the caregivers that it was her kitten who was responsible for the incident. This hilarious story proves lying isn't only an individual flaw in character.

The chapter includes a list of nonverbal red flags, as well as the description for each. In the next chapter, we'll discuss red flags that are verbal in the following chapter. A few of the red flags that are not verbal may be evident to everyone, but my aim is to ensure that this list of red flags is as complete as is possible. This list includes everything I've discovered when researching the subject. Before getting deeper into the details, however we'll discuss what that you should and shouldn't be doing when you're questioned by the person you're talking to. Here we go! ....

Koko was caught in the act of telling the lie of commission. There are three main types of lying: Commission, omission, and influence. Commission lies are kind that are made up by people who make them up. The lies of omission are vital details that someone deliberately doesn't disclose. The lies of influence, often known as character lies, are "not always untrue...but they attempt to give a false or inaccurate image" (Kasper, n.d.). A typical example of a character lies is when the employee is asked whether they have taken money from the company's coffee fund and they answer, "I've worked here 20 years!" It makes them seem like they're a decent employee, but that isn't a guarantee that they did not spend the money. Additionally, the sworn an oath which witnesses are required to take before they can stand on the stand as a witness at trial covers all three of these fables that I swear to speak the truth (covers the lies of commission) and the complete truth (covers lying of the omission) as well as nothing less than the truth (covers the lies of influence).

It's good to know that a majority of people are honest according to a report from 2021. Around 75% of the participants told lies between 0 and 2 times a day but only 6% those who participated averaged around 6 lies a each day. The majority of lies were small simple falsehoods. (Serota et al, 2022). Small white lies are often occasions told in order to ease the feelings of someone else. Other 90% of the lies are brought out as a result as a result of manipulating. They want that you behave or act to a way that's advantageous to them and certainly not for the person you are. If you think that someone has been lying about you, there are ways to deal with it. The trained interrogators are aware that lies are able to practice their speech and actions, but they rarely practice their bodies. They keep track of which types of questions trigger the biggest alarms (TED 2011, 2011). This is something you can try, as well.

Pay attention first to the person's "baseline" conduct. That is, look at the way they speak in a calm state and they have no reason to believe they are lying. Inquire about them in a way that they'd not have a reason to lie and observe their body expressions (Mishra 2014). These should be legitimate questions for that specific individual. What amount of eye contact does they offer to you? Not enough, too much or an amount that feels comfortable (to your eyes)? Most importantly, how much blinking is it? What's the body language they use when they're seated ....Are the legs extended or drawn closer to their bodies? Are they crossing their legs? Are their legs, feet or bodies turned toward the exit? Are the arms crossed? Do their hands feel relaxed and have some space between them, or are they bouncing? Are they very fidgety (do you tap your finger or bounce their feet on their feet?) Do they sit back, or are they moving toward the side? Do they rub their faces or neck? When you've gathered what they are doing while they seem at relaxed, look for any changes from their normal behavior.

Ask the tough questions. When you're asking these questions make sure you remain at peace and unaffected by the circumstances. Maintain your the voice and your the body language affable...Don't move your arms around or place the hands of your hips on the floor (it appears to be a sign of judgment). Be careful not to over-aggressive, since the opposite is true according to an expert investigator Pamela Meyer (TED, 2011). If you feel threatened will either do one of four things...They'll be unable to focus, get rid of then become more aggressive or even enter "denial lockdown". This is when they are compelled to believe in their lies regardless of how absurd they may appear. If they exhibit any of these four patterns that they aren't cooperating with them. Keep a positive relationship with the person. You may come across a time where you're furious at someone you think may have acted in a wrong way. It could be a family member who took funds from you, or someone in your relationship who was cheating against you. It's your opinion that they've committed immoral acts untrustworthy, apathetic, and most importantly terrible. It's difficult to maintain a civil relationship with their behavior. If you're angry at the moment, you should make sure to take time away from yourself in order to be calm and centered. This isn't straightforward, but the reality is that if doubt them while being emotional They'll likely be more deceitful to you or become aggressive for the need to protect themselves, and might even speak ill-omfussively towards the person you are. This isn't the result you're looking forward to. If you are able to let go of your feelings and ask those questions you'd like to learn, and you do it with calmness, it will lead closer to the reality. Then you can decide if you're going to forgive the person or end the friendship/relationship. This is extremely difficult or even impossible when you're not able to distinguish the difference between fiction and fact (Williams 2021).

If you're about to start with your questions, remember that how you approach these questions will make people feel extremely slammed or not. Be sure to avoid starting your question by asking "why" or "why not" unless you're hoping to make the person's brows rise. Use words which create a greater psychological barrier from the offensive behaviour. As an example Instead of asking "Why did you steal your cash?" ask "What made you choose to spend the cash?" (Imke, 2019) or "Do you have any idea what the source of the money might be?" Instead of "Why is it that you're late for the office?" try "How was your day getting to the office?" and instead of "Did you label Joe an"*sshole?" say "Did you perhaps say something rude to Joe in frustration?" Here's one last example...Instead of "Are you being a cheater on him?" say "Do you know why some people may think that you're cheating on him?" The way you pose your questions will help to maintain a positive relationship with the person you are asking questions that leads to better information. This gives them the chance to people to open up (Williams 2021). This doesn't mean that they'll however, you've provided them with an opportunity to try.

If you think someone might be not telling the truth then you could try asking the person an "bait query". Bait questions are scenario-based question which sounds similar to "Is there a reason? ...". Here are two instances. Let's suppose that there was a theft from your office and you think Joe Shmoe has something to be involved in the incident. Then, you ask him "Is there a reason people would claim to have seen me in my work space?" Now, it's an hypothetical query. Nobody actually said they were in your office However, you'd like to know his response to the question.

If he didn't visit your office and ought to have been there, the answer is "no". If he does take part in the incident, he'll begin to be concerned about the people who may have seen the man. It's likely to irritate the nerves of his body, and he may even come up with some excuse as to reasons he went to your workplace. If he's trying to hide something, it's possible to detect the red flags. To illustrate the second type of a bait-question Consider that your colleagues were involved in a conflict you have to figure out what the source of the situation is. It is your job to question two colleagues and the witnesses in a separate manner. You can ask "Is there a reason that the other witnesses would say differently than you've told me?" Hopefully, they'll be able to see that it's better to get their input, instead of having someone else reveal that they did the wrong thing and then lied about the incident (Price 2013, 2013). If they're telling the truth you shouldn't have a problem in answering the inquiry.

When you think of questions you'd like to be answered, create open-ended questions. This is a type of question where people are required to provide the answers themselves, instead of having choices to pick from. Think about this...You are asking Linda "Did you get your candy?" She says "no". It was an simple lie she could fabricate. She just had to speak one word and not give it much thinking. It makes lying more difficult for them. Remember this, also. ..."Liars tend to discover what they have already known, which is why asking open-ended questions force them to recall details that did not occur." In this case suppose you believe Joe Shmoe has been leaving at work in the morning. Instead of asking "Did you go to early Yesterday?" ask "When did you go to work last night?" or "What were your circumstances when you were able to leave work on the last day?"

In the course of your interaction, search for red flags that are clustered. These will likely appear in the first five seconds after every question. After that, they may not be visible for some time. The mere presence of a red flag might not be a sign of anything. But, two plus red flags the same time can indicate that they could have lied to you. So, look a bit deeper. Take heed...Some of what an untruthful person tells you will actually be truthful, so only pay attention to their claims that are accompanied by warning signs. So, do not be caught up trying to keep an eye on how many times you believe they're honest and you'll be overloaded (Digiday 2016, 2016).

This seems a little like a dance isn't it? Remember, like any other thing, you'll become more proficient with time and repetition. So, let's begin to get started...The below are the non-verbal indicators to be looking for:

1. Does their blinking speed vary?

A typical blink rate ranges between 16 to 20 blinks per minute. In stressful circumstances and with heavy mental load result in our blink rate to rise (Korda and others. 2021). Finding an effective lie can be mentally demanding, therefore it's a red signal. How can lying cause an enormous mental load? The reason is that the brain of a lying person is required to perform a variety of tasks all at once. In the first place, it must stop them from telling that they are telling the truth. Also, they must come up with the possibility of a plausible falsehood. In addition, they need to attempt to manage their body in order in order to look honest. It is also necessary to attempt to remember the lie they made up or any other lie they previously told that may conflict with the latest lie. In addition, they need to be attentive to their listeners in order to determine whether they are convincing the lies, at which time their blink speed could be reduced or cease for a few seconds depending on how they judge the situation (Rouse 2020). Another thing to note is that this warning alone isn't enough to conclude they're in fact lying. If they believe that you don't think they are lying, it can cause them to anxiety (thus an increase in blinks). Therefore, you should look out for other alarms.

2. If you're close enough to know Do their pupils dilate?

The pupils are enlarged. This is triggered when we encounter something we enjoy (wow they're so gentle to see!) or when we encounter things that make us feel scared. Also, it usually indicates the stress of our minds. The act of lying can cause fear and excessive mental stress. That's why pupils dilation is an indicator of a problem (Schafer 2019, 2019).

3. Are they staring at you in a way that is more than their normal?

If someone has been lying, they may be able to give you excessive eye contact. It could be an insidious effort to keep their eyes at you to determine whether you're being a victim of their lies. This could also be an intentional demonstration of their part...they might believe in the commonly held belief that lies aren't looking at you with a straight face. This is why they will stare at you in a bid to deflect this presumed dead-end. Imagine that someone is crying out loud or going wild. They're looking around, or putting their face in a mask. They're looking everywhere but focused on your. A third person is also having a meltdown and is going crazy and they are giving the impression of having lots in the way of contact. Who is deceiving? Most likely, the first one is real. When they're in this mindset it doesn't matter if they're gazing at you and don't even have the space within their minds to think whether you like what you think about the person. They could have something to hide from you.

#4 Do they avoid eye contact (unlike their norm)?

It is also known as "eye blocking" It could appear like one of the following...They speak something, and then look downwards or outwards a bit too long. It's a lot more than what you would have noticed in the normal behavior. They will say "no" and close their eyes in the same time however their eyes are closed for slightly longer than an ordinary blink. They apply their hand on their foreheads to form an obstruction for their eyes. They press on the bridge of their noses with the eyes shut. They scratch their eyes. They are simply able to shut their eyes. or, they stare straight at you, but lower than they do in their normal behavior. Someone who is deceiving use their subconscious eye blocking in order to block other people from seeing the sensitive details. Also, it is used to shield themselves from seeing the impact their deceitful actions have upon others. (Janine Driver "Reading Body Language"). Keep in mind that they are "red flags" rather than "lie indications". The closing of eyes by itself without any other red flags, is likely not a sign of blocking eyes however, it could be a reflection. In order to recollect things that don't come to our minds, we are likely to keep our eyes closed. The result is that visual stimulation decreases which allows our brains to concentrate on memory (Reeve 2019, 2019).

#5 Which direction are they looking?

Many people tend to look towards the same direction the dominant hand. Watch if you be aware of this within you. This is something that we all do in our minds. Someone who's in the process deceiving you could look away to their other aspect, and you should be aware of this warning sign (Williams 2021).

#6 Are their eyes flitting fast throughout the room?

The eyes that blink indicate they are deceiving. The person may be feeling trapped in the present and seeking a way to get out (Williams 2021).

7. Do they display their tongue for only a single second?

It can appear like lip licking. It's used for many different motives. If you're in a relationship the term usually refers to the person is interested. It could also indicate that someone is trying to appear attractive. It also plays the potential to be a factor in deceit. It is well-known that lying can make people feel anxious and uncomfortable as well as causes our mouths to dry (when the limbic system is putting our body in a state of fight or flight the body reserves fluids to our sweat glands and causes our mouths to dry) (Maxfield 2020). The act of putting your tongue out could also mean that someone doesn't believe what they've just stated. Also, we're searching for a group of negative signs, since the appearance of tongue could mean that they're not certain that what they stated was actually true.

#8 Does the person pause for to long prior to answering the inquiry?

It may be a quiet silence or a silence that is spoken. A lot of us say "Uuuuuuum" to complete the gap between words spoken while we are thinking of what else to say.

It can also buy lying time as well. You ask an issue, only to have them stare at you for a fraction of a moment too long before responding. An extended pause may indicate they're contemplating a falsehood (or perhaps trying to recall an idea they had in a previous time). It could also be a sign that they're not telling what they're planning to say. Therefore, take note of the words they use following this time of pause. Take care when you see this warning sign, however it is true that we require some time to respond to some concerns. Like, "Where were you on the 11th of March?" A person would have to take time to contemplate this question. If they stop when asked a question such as this, it's an indication of a problem: "Did you take my cash?" They don't need time to consider the solution in the event that they're truthful. If you are convinced that they're the ones responsible and you suspect that they are, then inquire "Is there a reason that someone observed you taking money from my wallet or purse?" If they're innocent They're likely to not answer and seem slightly confused about why someone will tell you this. If they're lying, this could prompt them to consider people who may have observed them and then told them about the incident. If this is the case it will trigger some pause. You should only use this method when your instinct says they have done it. If you do not, you may end up ruining an important relationship.

#9 Do they appear be losing the ability to speak?

It's similar to number 8. In this instance it is the case that the person attempts to speak, but is unable to find the appropriate word. Some people may even stutter. The reason for this is that they're worried about their situation. "They're trying but failing to determine how to proceed in the discussion." In the event that you observe this, it could be that the person might be planning to tell you something have already done so, or may have already made a false statement to you, or may be contemplating whether or not to reveal the truth or not (Williams 2021). Reminder...These aren't definitive evidence of fraud, but signals to alert you to look deeper (I recognize. I enjoy beating the dead horse).

#10 Do they put a mask on their mouths?

It is also known as blocking the mouth. It is when they put one or both hands toward their mouths. There are several reasons for people to mouth block. It may be that they don't really want to be asked the question or are subconsciously seeking to prevent them from speaking the truth. This is also a cover to cover up a lie that the person told. Additionally, they could mouth the block when you make a comment that they don't like, or even if they consider your words offensive (Williams 2021).

#11 Do they kiss their faces after answering the answer?

Be aware of a tug in their lips or around their ears or scratching their eyebrows, nose or forehead. If you're asking them questions that cause stress, their brains go to fight or flight. The organs of the lungs, the heart and the major muscles they'll have to endure and leaves the less vital parts that make up the human physique (like the ears, and other parts of the facial area) without blood. The "capillaries located in the places where blood is left get damaged and cause a feeling of coldness or itching." This is why there's pulling and scratching (Reeve 2019, 2019).

#12 Do you have a fake smile?

"Many people have a type of fake smile while they are lying" (Williams 2021). It's an unconscious muscle of the mouth that makes it appear more convincing. The smile conveys that everything is fine and the person is sincere because individuals don't smile when they know there's something wrong. The smile could be wide smile or even a tiny, Mona Lisa smile. Eyes won't be at all affected by the fake smile. That's right it won't cause an enlargement of the eye's corners or a squirting up on the tip of your nose. Beware of this.

#13 Are there grooming signs?

Grooming moves are a method to get rid of the the energy associated with deceit anxiety. You can look for signs like changing glasses, cleaning glasses making sure earrings are straight, adjusting the tie, pulling hair forward or pulling it behind ear, rubbing the body or head areas, picking fingersnails, making adjustments to the hat or pulling the sleeves up. Organising items or cleaning up areas are all thought to be grooming actions. Every move counts as being a red flag (Reeve, 2019,).

#14 When should they make use of hand gestures?

Watch out for people whose hands remain still when they speak. It's not an innate feature. A deceiving person is likely to talk with hands in a still position and then gesture their hands once they've spoken. However, a sincere person will tend to make gestures while they're speaking, or before beginning to talk. Experts in body language Traci Brown says that this is due to the cognitive load that lies creates can trigger the brain to defer the commands to regulate hand gestures (Jalili 2019, 2019).

#15 Can they make gestures using both hands?

According to a study conducted in 2015 that a person lying makes use of the hands of both hands 40 percent of the time as opposed to 25 percent of the time when truth-tellers are in the room (Perez-Rosas and co. (2015)).

#16 Have they hidden their hands from you?

"Clenched hands or closed palms...indicate the presence of restraint" (Meyer, n.d.). The suspects might not be giving you all the information but they may be feeling smug about their relationship with the way you present yourself. They're subconsciously preventing your eyes from their hands because they perceive that you are a danger. Maybe it's because they fear you might reveal something they're trying to conceal. By keeping their hands away from view sends the wrong message, whereas having them exposed to everyone; the message is "I do not have

anything to hide and I'm not an enemy".
Be sure to watch the palms of your palms.

#17 Are they putting some distance or wall
between you and them?

In a state of alert, our natural tendency is
to shield those areas that are vulnerable
to attack. Thus, an obnoxious person when
in this mode will seek to get more distance
between them and you as you could pose
a risk to the other. It is possible to see
through the deceit. It is possible that they
are consciously protecting their throat,
chest and head or stomach. It is
accomplished through consciously cross
their arms in front of the chest while
laying their clasped hands on their laps (in
in front of their abdomens) and cradling
their computer, clipboard and so on. on
their chests, or securing their necks by
putting their hands on it. (Williams, 2021).
There are politicians who clutch their
podiums or pressed on the. It is normal to

be just a couple of inches from it. If you spot these, they're probably employing their podiums as an obstruction between them and their viewers (Rouse 2020). What is the reason they decide to use this method? This is a red flag. Be aware of the feet of your guests. When they're sitting with their legs cross between their ankles? Are they moving their feet to the side, away from your? Are they pointing toward the exit? The person feels unsafe and is looking to get out (Meyer, n.d.).

#18 D0 do they give an instant shrug or single shoulder shrug? True shrugs show that the person isn't aware or doesn't want to. They're easy to recognize and are accompanied by both shoulders. They can last from 1 1/2 to 1 minute. Avoid the quick shrug, or the shrug with one shoulder. The person you are dealing with isn't trying to assist you and the way they shrug is a sign that you're in trouble (Meyer, n.d.).

#19 Do they clean their throats or do they swallow vigorously?

If your query creates anxiety in the person this can be manifested as dry throat and mouth. Check the Adam's Apple area to see if swallowing is occurring, as well as listen for a airy cough or a clear in the throat. The next step is important...You're checking to see whether this happens prior to the time they respond, since it's warning signs. If it happens immediately after answering to the question, it's most likely due to speaking that caused their throat and mouth dry. So, don't worry about the behavior (Reeve 2019, 2019).

#20 Are they able to nod their heads "yes" while they're saying "no" (or in reverse)?

The most common way to spot this is in situations where a person who is deceitful is offering a short "yes" as well as "no" response. The reason for this is due to the fact that you caught them in the wrong way with your query. They didn't have time to formulate an effective, deceitful response (Williams 2021). Here's an example...Let's suppose you're having the chance to host a potluck in your workplace where you want to ask your coworker about their opinion about the cheese dish. They're now contemplating whether or not you prepared it, or whether someone else was close to them, and aren't looking to hurt anyone's sentiments. They respond by saying, "It's good," however, their head is move a bit to the side when they speak the words. It could be that the dish isn't as good.

#21 Do they show the quick "duping joy" smile?

The people who don't like lying are not likely to experience the joy when they are duped. The more manipulative lying liars who feel the joy of ripping off one another and then getting away by doing the resulting smear. The smile appears to be a fake that's not in the place. The most frightening example of this can be seen during an interview with the convicted killer Diane Downs. Her display of delight in the duper was out of context and terrifying. Duper's joy displays tend to be as apparent. Be on the lookout for smiles that look to be out of place.

#22 Are they looking at the partner before or during a speech?

It is also known as"a "confirmation look". Expert in body language Chase Hughes uses the acronym CRASH to explain the reason people might use this. First, they're looking for confirmation from their accomplice...either the head nod or an "mm-hmm" or "yeah" to provide them with an encouragement or to back them up. Then, they're searching for Relief. Perhaps they are hoping that their partner will do the job their duties, and they are able to relax some. They also want approval from their companion. They're like trying to figure out, "How am I doing?" Fourthly, they could be searching for an idea from their partner. They're in the middle of a speech however they aren't sure what to do next and they're looking for their accomplice to give them their next words. In the end, they're searching for assistance. They believe that the things are going wrong which is why they're trying to convince their companion to keep working for the sake of their family or amend their statement. Again, remember that 1 red flag alone is not enough to conclude they're lying (Truecrimeworkshop.com).

#23 What is an inappropriate way to display comfort?

Let's suppose there's an incident of fraud within the company employees are being probed. While he is being questioned, Joe Shmoe clasps his hands and spreads his hands out towards the front in order to relax his lower back. It's a very serious thing to do that is why it's unusual for any person to be relaxed enough to stretch at this time. This could mean that Joe wants to seem relaxed with the idea that a person who is innocent would not have any reason to be worried. Imagine that Chloe Shmoee accuses her boyfriend of unfaithfulness He lets out a swig. This is also a bit inappropriate to do so at the present time. Perhaps it is a method to downplay the seriousness of the statements and concerns raised by Chloe.

Incredibly, there's an illness known as psychogenic belching where people burp repeatedly at a rapid rate when anxious (the word "psychogenic" signifies that the reason is a psychological issue, not physical). The cause is the condition known as aerophagia. It's characterized by excessive swallowing of air. The normal way to swallow is some air while eating, swallowing or speaking, but the condition of aerophagia elevates it to the next dimension. It may occur prior to any increase in anxiety in the midst of a full-blown panic attack or when the individual is calmed (Folk 2022).

#24 Does the anchor point show moving or fidgeting?

Be aware of these movements particularly after asking a an explicit question. Anchor points refer to any point where the body's physique and a solid object. As an example, when you're sitting down, your butt will be in contact with the seat. Does their weight shift into the chair? If they lean to the side, their back is touching the rear of the chair. Does the chair make a turn by bending their back? The feet are usually the anchor point. Are they bouncing either their legs or feet? Do they dance their feet? If they have their hands resting on the table, will they begin tapping their hands? Do they begin engaging their hands? Are they able to move their hands towards their laps? Do they take out the pencil and begin twirling the pencil? Do they shake their heads downwards, backwards, or even to the side? Find any small signs that resemble these. The anchor point is moved in a subconscious way to alleviate any discomfort due to anxiety. fidgeting can help let go of the anxiety-inducing energy. In reality, a honest person may feel anxious due to having to respond to questions, particularly if they're someone they've never met. However, someone who is deceitful will experience the most stress from being required to work hard to avoid making errors that could expose them. However there is a lot of pressure for the deceitful person is higher, and you'll probably see more alarms coming from those who are deceived. Consider every movement of the anchor point and fidgeting as red flags (Reeve 2019, 2019). Note...Some falsely informed people believe that lying people fidget. Therefore, they'll deliberately freeze their bodies in order to prevent this. Be aware of the person who appears to be unnaturally quiet even when they're conversing, higher than the normal manner of behavior. The person could be trying to cover something up from you.

Do you think your silence causes you stress?

When someone has finished the answer to the question You should let them wait at least 3 minutes. Keep your eyes on them for this time. Someone who is deceitful will be in a state of anxiety but this period of silence may agitate the suspect even more. The silence could make them add "more relevant details" (Imke 2019, 2019). It is important to take a pause after each question. You should also be watching their movements throughout every break.

#26 Do they notice a difference in the way they breathe?

Like we said earlier the stress of lying may trigger the "fight-or-flight" mode to come on. Heart rate increases that causes an increase in breath. When a person begins to breath faster, this is undoubtedly a warning sign. The person may also be able to subconsciously take their breath in for a few seconds. This can happen when one is engaged in a significant mental load (such the ones that lying can create). For a person to recognize this alert for a deep breath, or an exaggerated breath (Williams 2021).

#27 Have they made a shift in the way they speak?

Look out for the red flags They will notice that the pitch of their voice gets higher. They begin speaking slower (it helps them to save time). Then they suddenly begin to speak louder. Their words diminish from normal to whispers or silence (suggesting they're giving up on the lie since they aren't convinced that it's effective) (Williams 2021).

Do they begin sweating?

Do you develop tiny sweaty beads around their lips or forehead? It's because the person in question is putting such a massive pressure on their body that they appear calm and normal (Williams 2021).

Do they appear happy if they see a change of topic?

If you think someone lies about you, consider changing the topic. Are they happy? (Mishra (2015)) If they do it could be because they feel they've been granted a break from the lies they're committing. The same is true for when they pay attention to their body language in the event that an outside force creates an interruption in the interview (i.e. rain drips off the ceiling, or you receive the phone, etc.).

#30 Are the two faces on their sides displaying different feelings?

If all is side of the up and down, both sides your face are the same or display similar emotions. Watch out for the one whose face makes their face appear oddly. This is because they don't believe in something and the body doesn't totally commit to the expression...They're not fully moving around (Navarro 2008.).

#31 Do they soothe themselves?

Self-soothing is a process that occurs subconsciously in people in times of stress (and how does lying contribute to anxiety? You got it...anxiety). The person might rub their upper back of their neck or hug themselves, stretch their thighs or arms or shake their hands.

#32 Do their faces turn either flush or pale?

In this case, anxiety is the cause of this. In the fight or flight state, it results in blood flowing elsewhere and leave the skin with either greater fluid (flush) or less (pale) that is normal.

#33 Does there seem to be a lack of mirroring?

When there's trust and respect for each other mirroring of body movements is likely to take place, either conscious or in a subconscious way. As an example, two people tend to lean forward while keeping their hands placed on the table either leaning back or forward. The two end up leaning back and putting their heads into their hands, or crossed their legs. If you believe someone may be lying it will show an absence of mirroring. This is because of the absence of a connection and the inability to engage. Make a slight adjustment to the way you move your body to see if the other person are mirroring you. If they do not, it's unintentional (Williams 2021).

Don't forget to listen to your instinctive reactions. "A several studies indicate that your first instincts are far more immediate and most likely to be right. This is why...There are no facial expressions that is a lie. The face has 42 muscles on the facial muscles (43 in the case of counting the tongue) The muscles can be used for more than 10,000 expressions. In addition, each expression may take just one 5th of second, or lesser! This is too short for the brain to recognize and yet the unconscious can detect it. Therefore, if your instincts are warning you that a person is fraudulent, consider it warning signs (Reeve 2019, 2019).

Author's note: Just one more item before we move on to the subject of non-verbal cues...When I was in the company of some loved friends and acquaintances heard that I had written my book, they inquired whether I'd heard of "eye accessibility". The concept was taught in the field of body language. It was believed that looking up or to the right was an indication of lying. 3 separate studies of eye access have shown that this method isn't effective. If you're thinking why it's not on my red flag list it's because of this (Wolchover 2012).

Chapter 11: Secrets Of Lie Detecting

(VERBAL RED FLAGS)

Certain researchers have claimed that identifying verbal signals is more efficient than reading nonverbal signals. Therefore, now knowing what are nonverbal signals to be looking for, let us fill your toolbox further by incorporating verbal cues.

Finding the truth is crucial, and scientists are working on the use of ways to spot deceit from the 1970s. This is just one of the research studies that proved to be enlightening...In the year 2016, researchers employed the software they developed to assist researchers analyze over 1,000 claims made by two executives who were accused of committing fraud at work. It was discovered that the "fraudulent statements tend to be longer and more specific than their truthful ones" in addition to being much more "fuzzy" in addition to being "uncertain". In addition, their false statements were more positive in comparison to their honest ones. (Association for Psychological Science, 2016). Their lies were more elaborate? They employed more positive language while lying? It may seem odd, this is precisely why results from research like this can be so important.

In the case of nonverbal red flags, it's best to be searching for two plus red signals quick in succession (5 minutes is a great guideline). You can also look for 2 plus red flags for each query. If there are greater the number of red flags (verbal as well as non-verbal) you spot more likely of the individual being misleading, therefore you should dig a little further. I'll be specific about this...Listen to the statements of the individual completely. Do not stop listening even if you've noticed several suspicious signs. Be attentive to what they speak. If you're not sure on something they've mentioned Ask them to explain. You'll be able to get a better grasp of their meaning as well as they'll think you're respectful to the person, which makes them talk to you in a more relaxed manner. We'll now take a look at some of the verbal dangers.

#1 Do they the distancing of language?

This kind of speech is utilized by those trying to create a formal "distance" between them with an occasion. They use it to conceal they are deceiving themselves as they believe lying as not savory and is in direct contradiction with their principles (DBpedia 2019). In the case of others, distancing words is used consciously and deliberately to deceive you into ignoring the truth.

What is this language that distancing sounds like? The answer is that it does not allow self-referencing. This is possible in three distinct methods. One method is to employ"passive" voice. In other words, instead of telling the audience "I put the safe unlocked" They use the phrase "the safe was left unlocked". Instead of "I knocked Grandma's cherished porcelain statue off the shelf " They use the phrase "it was knocked off the shelves". Instead of "we drove the car off the edge" instead, they state "the car fell off the edge". The idea is obvious. Distancing words are used to keep from taking responsibility for the incident. A person who is honest usually uses the word "I" in describing the actions they took during an event. Here's an example of the way the truthful person can be able to explain the events that occurred. ..."I arrived home at 5:45. Just as I was getting ready lock my front door I heard an explosion at the inside. My pets aren't my thing and so I was walking through the exterior of my home, taking a look at the windows. This is when I noticed my television had gone. I made a call to the police immediately." The suspect employed the word "I" 7 times as well as "my" three times. A deceiving person might not use any of the self-referencing verbs (I myself, me myself, my we, ourselves ours, ourselves, or us). They could be trying to avoid drawing focus to themselves ("Distancing the language" 2022).

Another way to prevent self-referencing is by using "the was able to understand you" pronoun, instead in place of "I". As an example, instead "I was in a rush to go to the appointment with my doctor, and I didn't secure the safe before leaving" or "well it happens when you're in rush and need to get somewhere else by the exact time then you don't remember everything you're required to accomplish, therefore it's true that the safe was not locked".

The final method to avoid this is to just remove pronouns which would typically be used, such as in the next example. The following statement was given by a man who claims that his wife's death was accidental: "I picked up the gun and cleaned it. I moved it to my left hand, to retrieve the rod to clean it. The trigger was hit by something. The gun fired off striking my wife." The man used "I" throughout the initial sentence and then used "my" within the second phrase, however notice how the sentence in the second paragraph begins by using the word "moved". This way it was avoided that he took directly the responsibility for the actions of shooting the gun. Additionally, he decided to use "the left hand" instead of "my left hand" as many people will be able to say. The man also stated that "something" was the reason for the trigger to activate this allowed him to not take responsibility for the trigger's failure to trigger. It's possible that this man was not able to acknowledge that he was responsible for death to his dear wife, or perhaps deliberately did the thing. It's either way, it's still an alarming warning sign (Clikeman 2012).

It's a final thing to consider when distancing a language. An unintentionally deceiving person could utilize "that" in place of "this" or "those" in place in place of "these" ("Distancing languages," 2022). It's more subtle distancing. The way in which the word "that" refer to the distance? If you were in front of your vehicle, you'd be saying, "This is mine." If, however, you were in a distance from it that you'd be required to show it off and say "That's mine there." Let's suppose an officer has summoned a murdered suspect to be questioned. The detective places a huge image of the weapon used in the crime (a big hunting knife) placed on a table the front of him. First, let's assume that the suspect looks briefly at the image, and after which he looks at the policeman and states "That's it's not mine." Then, let's suppose that the suspect takes the image to look it more attentively. In about two minutes, he puts the picture back on his desk and looks up at the policeman and states, "This isn't my knife." This is an insignificant difference however, in the first instance it is apparent that the suspect has place more distance between himself and the knife with his actions as well as the choice of phrases. The suspect is unable to even get himself to glance at the picture and even less take it home. It's an alarming sign because the person who is guilty tends to attempt to distance themselves from them and the situation. Here's a concrete example that shows this diaspora from the language. This is a quote by the president Bill Clinton in regards to Monica Lewinsky. Clinton said "I didn't have sexual relationships with this woman...Ms. Lewinsky." It would have been possible to say he stated "with her" but instead decided to use "with this woman".

2. Is there "severity in softening" in their language?

Severity softening has a lot to do with to the distancing of language. And people don't just use it to conceal our identity. In the case of burial, for example. loved one can be emotionally challenging and so, instead of saying "We will be burying Grandma next Saturday" it could be "Grandma is going to lay to rest on Saturday." The use of severity softening can help to make a psychological distinction from the harsh real life. It is a factor in the act of lying too. Look at statements of two distinct people. Person A states, "I wouldn't take it." Person B states, "I don't steal." Which one sounds like they're speaking the truth? Someone who is in the process of being guilty will employ less harsh words, therefore, person A may reduce the seriousness of their offense. Another example of mildening the severity the severity of a crime: Someone who is guilty might claim, "I wouldn't do such an act," whereas an honest individual might state, "I didn't do it." (Academic, n.d.) The perpetrators of murder will utilize phrases such as "harm" as well as "hurt" while the family members of victims use terms that mean "kill" as well as "murder" (Note it is noted that Susan Smith said, "I don't want to hurt my children"). Families of victims are angry at the loss of their loved ones. Therefore, it's difficult to find phrases that diminish the seriousness of the offense. Other examples of severity softening the guilty party's words "warned" in place of "threatened", "bumped" instead of "hit", "missing" instead of "stolen" or "stolen" and "borrowed" and "picked picked up" as opposed to "stolen" (Clikeman 2012).

3. Do they not respond to your query?

You might, for instance, inquire, for instance "Do you have any idea why my weight isn't there?" You're met with silence or something similar to, "You've got the wrong person. Ask Mike," and they aren't able to answer your query. This doesn't necessarily mean that the person is guilty but this is a red flag. Also, pay attention to those who give an appearance of responding. As an example, suppose you asked a worker about the importance of data deleted. The following is their response. ..."I always try backing to my laptop and then put the papers away every at night prior to going to bed. On Tuesday, I made the decision to save my data onto the network drive, and began organizing my files into my drawer at work. It was also necessary to lock the client list inside the Office safe." The staff spoke many things in their response however did they provide an exact answer? No. They told me, "I try to back to my computer...every every night." An answer that is definitive could have been "I have backed up my laptop computer." Also, they said, "I decided to copy my data" and not "I transferred my files." Finally they stated, "I...needed to lock the...list...in the...safe" and not "I put the list into the safe." This caustic kind of response can trick the reader into believing that they performed everything they mentioned and not even admitting they completed these things (Clikeman 2012).

4. Are they hesitant to speak up?

If someone doesn't want to respond to your inquiry They might respond with things like "I'm not sure if I'm best person to speak with regarding that" or "Gosh I'm not certain I'm qualified to answer this". It could be a sign of innocence However, it is important to think of it as a red signal and ask them additional questions (Reeve 2019.).

#5 Does the person you ask question using the "dodgeball"?

Here are a few examples of dodgeball-related questions: "Why do you ask?", "Why would you believe that I committed the crime?", "Why would I commit such a crime?", "Why would I do that to my family member?", "Do I look like a person who'd commit something like this?", and "Don't you think someone has been pretty dumb to swipe money out of their bank account?" When a person responds to a question by asking another one, it may be that they're merely making a purchase of time in the process of thinking up the answer. However, they could also be trying to determine what you are aware of before revealing an information that may reveal their lies (Imke 2019, 2019).

Someone who is deceived could reply by asking an irrelevant query to gain time. Imagine that you work for an office and there's the laptop you don't have a record for. The employee you inquire with asks to confirm if they have taken it and they reply by asking, "How much did it cost?" or "How old was it?" Does it matter what it cost, or the age of it? No. It was either a laptop or weren't. An honest person will say not at first and inquire further about it (Reeve, 2019,).

#6 Is the first sentence an unanswerable question?

Another strategy is to purchase time. Some examples are "That's an excellent to ask", "I'm glad you have asked me this", "I knew you wanted to have me ask this" And "That's an appropriate worry". It is important to ask them additional inquiries to find out the if they're merely being polite or actually wish to assist you (Reeve, 2019,).

#7 Can they respond with a reference statement?

The use of referrals allows the deceitful individual to seem to be cooperating by replying to you without having to repeat the lie. Susan Carnicero, former CIA security expert, says the following "It's difficult to admit that you've been lying or committed an error." Therefore an official spokesperson of an organisation might answer with a reference to the previous responses, for example "As we stated in our press announcement" ..." as well "Like we talked about on our quarterly conference call ..." (TDAmeritrade Institutional n.d.).

Referral statements can also be employed by a deceitful individual to establish credibility. This is done by referring you to somebody who is not you. As an example, "Ask him. He'll tell you." (Andreae, n.d.). That's what a true teller might say as well. If it's someone who's lying to you about that, they are aware that the person they're referring to will support them since they're working in cahoots. That's why it's known as a red signal. Keep in mind that you're searching for two or more red flags in a single question and red flags are just an indication to look a bit deeper.

#8 Will they answer the question with aggression?

If you inquire about someone's opinion, then they pop up in your throat saying something like, "I don't believe this!", it's a warning sign. This would spare everybody's time by simply answering the question. Instead, they're trying to make you feel that they're wrong for refusing to answer questions. They're attempting to take the pressure away from themselves and to your shoulders. Other examples include "Oh Please!", "Here we come again!", "Why don't you believe you?", "Is this an act of deceit?", "Are you asking everyone or myself?", "It's a somewhat rude question to ask this, don't you think?", and "Why do you waste my time in the question?" Note that their anger could be directed towards someone else, and not only yourself. That's still an indication of a problem (Digiday 16th, 2016). Sometimes rather than making people feel guilty about making a request, the perpetrators will try to undermine your credibility. In this case, they might ask things like "How how long has it been since you started this work?", "Do you know anything about the business?", and even "Is this an elaborate ploy?" (Reeve, 2019).

www.ingramcontent.com/pod-product-compliance
Lightning Source LLC
Chambersburg PA
CBHW051728020426
42333CB00014B/1209